# Pancreatic Cytopathology

# ESSENTIALS IN CYTOPATHOLOGY SERIES

*Dorothy L. Rosenthal, MD, FIAC, Series Editor*

**Editorial Board**

*Syed Z. Ali, MD*
*Douglas P. Clark, MD*
*Yener S. Erozan, MD*

# David C. Chhieng, MD, MBA, MSHI

Department of Pathology, University of Alabama at Birmingham, Birmingham, Alabama

# Edward B. Stelow, MD

Department of Pathology, University of Virginia, Charlottesville, Virginia

# Pancreatic Cytopathology

Foreword by Michael W. Stanley, MD

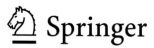 Springer

David C. Chhieng, MD, MBA, MSHI
Professor of Pathology
Department of Pathology
University of Alabama at Birmingham
Birmingham, AL 35249-7331
USA

Edward B. Stelow, MD
Assistant Professor
Department of Pathology
University of Virginia
Charlottesville, VA 22908-0214
USA

*Series Editor*
Dorothy L. Rosenthal, MD, FIAC
Professor of Pathology, Oncology, and Gynecology and Obstetrics
The Johns Hopkins Medical Institutions
Director of Pathology
The Johns Hopkins Bayview Medical Center
Baltimore, MD 21287
USA

Library of Congress Control Number: 2006940467

ISBN: 978-0-387-68946-3          e-ISBN: 978-0-387-68947-0

Printed on acid-free paper.

9 8 7 6 5 4 3 2

springer.com

To our families, teachers, and friends for their
love and support.

# Foreword

Diagnosis by cytologic means is what the mathematicians would describe as elegant; the methods are often simple but richly nuanced, while the results can be profound though succinctly stated. Tiny samples atraumatically obtained are at the heart of both the elegance and the difficulties of this subspecialty.

Following initial successes of traditional exfoliative cytology, further applications were long constrained by the fact that few body surfaces present themselves for direct collection of exfoliated cells. Thus, it was inevitable that advances in nonoperative evaluations for specific body sites would be accompanied by expansions in cytologic diagnosis. Hence the proliferation of sampling methods with techniques the same as their names, including brushing, washing, lavage, and aspiration.

Examples come readily to mind. One of the most dramatic bursts in cytodiagnosis happened in the 1980s, when deep-lung sampling by bronchoalveolar lavage (BAL) arrived at about the same time as the AIDS pandemic. Frequent and often repeated diagnosis of CMV and pneumocystis quickly led to numerous such samples being submitted to many laboratories. These now common infectious agents and this new technique were highly suited to rapid evaluation of AIDS patients.

The rapid rise of fine needle aspiration occurred at about the same time, at least on this side of the Atlantic. Although not really new, the explosion in its use had awaited both clinical acceptance and adequate training for a critical mass of pathologists. This history has been well recorded by others.

Cytology is now entering yet another era of dramatic growth. The new field of endoscopic ultrasound-guided fine needle aspiration (EUS-FNA) has brought together several elements: considerable recent advances in our knowledge of pancreatobiliary pathology; specially trained gastroenterologists comfortable with these nontraditional anatomic projections; pathologists with skill in surgical pathology and cytopathology of this complex part of the body; and the information technology needed to process the detailed images that result from high-frequency ultrasound.

The cytopathologist faces new and complex interpretive issues associated with characteristics of this method and the resulting samples. First, many of the malignancies are well-differentiated adenocarcinomas and must be distinguished from abundant gastric and duodenal mucosal samplings with their own attendant range of nonneoplastic alterations. Second, identification of mucinous contaminants from the upper gastrointestinal lumen can make it very difficult to identify the often low-grade mucinous neoplasms found in this area. Other cells that require special attention were previously described, but can take on new significance in this context. These include hepatocytes, adrenal cortical tissue, and ganglion cells.

Clinical applications of this method are expanding as rapidly as practitioners can be trained. This, in turn, requires that the community of diagnostic cytopathology mount a similar response. The current book by Drs. Stelow and Chhieng will fill a yawning gap in this important literature from both the pedagologic and practice points of view. These two investigators are not only active in this exciting new application of cytodiagnosis; they have collectively contributed some of its most important investigational advances.

Pathologists who do not currently examine pancreatic cytology samples and EUS-FNA material will shortly be called upon to do so. This new book will do much to smooth the way.

*Michael W. Stanley, MD*
St. Paul, MN
May 2007

# Series Preface

The subspecialty of cytopathology is 60 years old and has become established as a solid and reliable discipline in medicine. As expected, cytopathology literature has expanded in a remarkably short period of time, from a few textbooks prior to the 1980's to a current library of texts and journals devoted exclusively to cytomorphology that is substantial. *Essentials in Cytopathology* does not presume to replace any of the distinguished textbooks in Cytopathology. Instead, the series will publish generously illustrated and user-friendly guides for both pathologists and clinicians.

Building on the amazing success of *The Bethesda System for Reporting Cervical Cytology*, now in its second edition, the *Series* will utilize a similar format including minimal text, tabular criteria and superb illustrations based on real-life specimens. *Essentials in Cytopathology* will, at times, deviate from the classic organization of pathology texts. The logic of decision trees, elimination of unlikely choices and narrowing of differential diagnosis via a pragmatic approach based on morphologic criteria will be some of the strategies used to illustrate principles and practice in cytopathology.

Most of the authors for *Essentials in Cytopathology* are faculty members in The Johns Hopkins University School of Medicine, Department of Pathology, Division of Cytopathology. They bring to each volume the legacy of John K. Frost and the collective experience of a preeminent cytopathology service. The archives at Hopkins are meticulously catalogued and form the framework for text and illustrations. Authors from other institutions have been selected on the basis of their national reputations, experience and enthusiasm for Cytopathology. They bring to the series complimentary viewpoints and enlarge the scope of materials contained in the photographs.

The editor and authors are indebted to our students, past and future, who challenge and motivate us to become the best that we possibly can be. We share that experience with you through these pages, and hope that you will learn from them as we have from those who have come before us. We would be remiss if we did not pay tribute to our professional colleagues, the cytotechnologists and preparatory technicians who lovingly care for the specimens that our clinical colleagues send to us.

And finally, we cannot emphasize enough throughout these volumes the importance of collaboration with the patient care team. Every specimen comes to us as a question begging an answer. Without input from the clinicians, complete patient history, results of imaging studies and other ancillary tests, we cannot perform optimally. It is our responsibility to educate our clinicians about their role in our interpretation, and for us to integrate as much information as we can gather into our final diagnosis, even if the answer at first seems obvious.

We hope you will find this series useful and welcome your feedback as you place these handbooks by your microscopes, and into your bookbags.

*Dorothy L. Rosenthal, M.D., FIAC*
Baltimore Maryland
drosenthal@jhmi.edu
July 15, 2004

# Contents

# 1
# Introduction to Pancreatic Cytopathology

The use of fine needle aspiration biopsy (FNA) and duct brushing and aspiration in the management of patients with pancreatic masses has been well established. These procedures are considered accurate and minimally aggressive for obtaining tissue diagnoses.

## Indications of Cytologic Sampling

The most common indication for cytologic sampling is to document malignancy in patients with malignant-appearing pancreatic masses on imaging. For patients with inoperable tumors, a tissue diagnosis can preclude unnecessary surgery and allow the initiation of chemotherapy and/or radiation therapy. For patients who are surgical candidates, a preoperative tissue diagnosis allows for the optimal planning of surgery.

The differential diagnosis for a pancreatic mass is extensive and comprises a wide spectrum of lesions, both non-neoplastic and neoplastic. It is not surprising, then, that another goal for pancreatic sampling is the determination of the nature of an "atypical" pancreatic lesion or mass identified on imaging. Cytologic findings can then guide subsequent management.

# Methods of Sampling

Methods of sampling generally include brushings or aspiration from within the common bile or pancreatic duct and FNA. Intraductal brushings and aspiration are performed using endoscopic retrograde cholangiopancreatography (ERCP) or percutaneous transhepatic cholangiography (PTC), which allow for the identification and sampling of ductal abnormalities such as strictures or dilatations. These procedures do not generally allow for the appreciation of a mass, per se, but are instead performed because of their interventional capabilities, such as the stenting of the ductal system.

Pancreatic masses can be aspirated intraoperatively either by palpation or direct visualization. More frequently, however, sampling is performed under image guidance. Transabdominal ultrasound (US) and computed tomography (CT) are the two preferred imaging techniques for percutaneous approach. Ultrasound allows for sampling of the lesion in real time; however, visualization of the target lesion can be impaired by intervening bowel and fat. Computed tomography provides better visualization and resolution but does not allow for the real-time identification of the needle tip during sampling.

In recent years, advances in technology have permitted the performance of FNA under endoscopic ultrasound (EUS) guidance. This procedure uses an echoendoscope, which consists of an endoscope with an attached ultrasound transducer on its tip. A curvilinear echoendoscope provides a 100° view parallel to the long axis of the scope that allows for continuous, real-time visualization of a needle as it punctures its target lesion. Endoscopic ultrasound–fine needle aspiration (EUS-FNA) also has the ability to sample small lesions that may not be seen by CT or conventional US and can better detect vascular and nodal involvement. A major disadvantage of EUS-FNA is that one must undergo considerable training to become proficient in this technique.

Needles used for FNA vary in caliber. Smaller needles, such as 20- to 25-gauge needles, are associated with fewer complications particularly if multiple passes are required. Tissue cores can be obtained when 18-gauge or larger needles are used, but such sampling is usually not necessary and may be associated with a higher risk of complications.

## Contraindications

There are few absolute contraindications to pancreatic FNA. They include uncorrectable bleeding diathesis and the lack of a safe access path. For patients undergoing EUS-FNA, the presence of gastrointestinal obstruction is an absolute contra-indication. The aspiration of uncooperative patients is also contraindicated because of increased risk of complications.

## Complications

Table 1-1 lists the possible complications of pancreatic FNA. In general, complications of FNA are infrequent (average, 2%) and tend to be mild, for example, vasovagal reaction, abdominal discomfort, and small hemorrhage. Mortal injury is exceedingly rare but can result from acute hemorrhagic pancreatitis or sepsis. Infectious complications are more common in patients with cystic lesions and, therefore, antibiotic prophylaxis is often given to patients with these

TABLE 1-1. Complications of pancreatic FNA.

Vasovagal reaction
Abdominal discomfort
Infectious complications—bacteremia and abscess (especially following the
   aspiration of cystic lesions)
Acute pancreatitis
Bile peritonitis
Hemorrhage
Bowel perforation (EUS-FNA)
Tumor seeding along needle tract (rare)

lesions. The risk of bowel perforation in patients undergoing EUS is very low and is comparable with that of standard endoscopy, which is less than 1%. Risk factors for perforation include an inexperienced operator, an elderly patient, and esophageal stricture. The potential for tumor seeding along the needle tract has raised concerns, particularly for patients with resectable tumors. Most studies, however, have shown no increased incidence of peritoneal seeding or any adverse changes in patient outcome following pancreatic FNA.

## Sample Preparation

It is important to keep in mind that optimal specimen preparation is the key for obtaining an adequate sample and the correct interpretation. It therefore may be best for aspirated material to be processed by cytology personnel. We recommend the following protocol:

1. Slides are labeled appropriately and placed on a smooth surface.

2. For each pass, aspirated material is expressed on the glass slides by forcing air into the needle through an attached air-filled syringe (Figure 1-1).

3. Both air-dried and alcohol-fixed smears are prepared.

4. The needle can then be rinsed in Hank's balanced-salt solution or other normal saline-based solutions for cell block preparations. The needle can also be rinsed in alcohol-based solution for the preparation of thin layer slides and/or cell block. Finally, as samples obtained by EUS-FNA are often bloody, we have made cell blocks by allowing bloody material to clot on a slide, scraping the clotted material into 10% neutral buffered formalin, and then processing by routine histology (Figure 1-2).

5. Air-dried smears can be stained with a modified Romanowsky method (e.g., Diff-Quik) for onsite assessment of specimen adequacy and a provisional or preliminary diagnosis can be made, if possible.

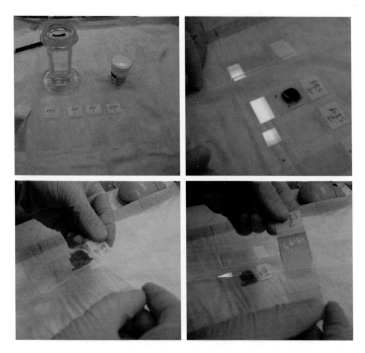

FIGURE 1-1. Slides are labeled appropriately and placed on a smooth surface. Aspirate is expressed on the glass slides by forcing air into the needle through an attached air-filled syringe. Smears are made by transferring a small amount of aspirate via the end of a clean glass slide onto another clean and labeled slide and smearing the aspirate to make a thin film on the labeled slide. The transfer slide is then discarded.

6. Additional samples can be obtained for ancillary studies such as flow cytometry and microbiologic culture, if deemed necessary.

Because blood may dilute the diagnostic materials and clot, obscuring the cellular details of the specimens, the optimal cytologic preparation should consist of as little blood as possible. Clotting can be minimized by obtaining and preparing the samples promptly. We prefer block preparation to liquid-based preparations because it allows for the ready use of

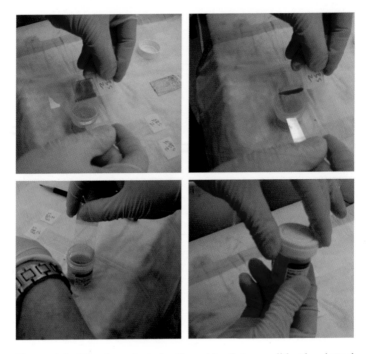

FIGURE 1-2. Bloody aspirate is allowed to clot on a slide; the clotted material is then scrapped, using another glass slide, into 10% neutral buffered formalin for subsequent processing of cell block.

immunocytochemistry and other special techniques and also can provide information about cellular architecture. In addition, background material can be lost with liquid-based preparations. Cyst fluid collected by aspiration can be sent for the analysis of relative viscosity, tumor markers, and pancreatic enzymes to assist with the distinction between non-neoplastic and neoplastic cysts.

Most authors agree that the presence of a cytologist during the procedure is beneficial. Major advantages include higher diagnostic yields and, potentially, reduced numbers of required passes. Patients can be spared the risk and unpleasantness of another procedure as well as the cost associated with it. In addition to assessing specimen adequacy onsite, the cytologist can also determine if additional material is needed for ancillary studies such as immunocytochemistry and flow cytometry. Immediate interpretation also enables pathologists to render preliminary diagnoses, which, in most cases, agree with final diagnoses, and allow clinicians to make timely referrals to appropriate specialists. Both clinicians and patients, however, should be warned that, in rare occasions, the final diagnosis may be different from the preliminary diagnosis when additional cytologic material becomes available for examination.

## Performance

The specificity of malignant diagnoses for pancreatic FNA approaches 100%, as most cytopathologists have high thresholds for diagnosing pancreatic neoplasia. On the contrary, early literature reported the sensitivity of pancreatic FNA for diagnosing malignancy to be as low as 50%. More recent reports demonstrate a much improved performance. For FNA performed percutaneously under CT or US guidance, the reported sensitivity ranges from 85% to 95% and for EUS-FNA, the reported sensitivity ranges from 75% to 95%. The improvement of sensitivity can likely be attributed to better diagnostic yields and the better recognition and application of diagnostic criteria. Such results are often derived from series that consist predominantly of the sampling of solid pancreatic lesions, however. When only cystic pancreatic lesions are considered, the sensitivity of FNA for detecting neoplasia falls dramatically, to as low as 60%.

Papers dealing with brushings and intraductal aspirations also report lower sensitivities for the diagnosis of pancreatic neoplasia, usually between 45% and 70%. Both sampling errors, due to the failure of neoplasms to shed diagnostic cells into the ducts, and interpretive errors, secondary to obscuring material or artifact, have been shown to contribute to the relatively low sensitivities.

TABLE 1-2. Causes of false-negative diagnoses.

Sampling errors
  Small lesions
  Difficult anatomic location
  Extensive fibrosis
  Extensive necrosis
  Excessive bleeding
  Operator's inexperience
Interpretative errors
  The underdiagnosis of well-differentiated or low-grade neoplasms
  Nonspecific cyst fluid findings
Obscuring factors and artifacts
  Excessive air drying
  Obscuring inflammation
  Obscuring necrotic debris
  Contamination by benign gastrointestinal epithelium (EUS-FNA)

False-positive diagnoses with FNA are rare and often are due to the overinterpretation of reactive epithelial atypia. False-negative results are not infrequent and range from 4% to 14% in most series. Table 1-2 lists the common causes of false-negative diagnoses. They include sampling error, the underinterpretation of well-differentiated or low-grade neoplasms, such as well-differentiated adenocarcinomas or acinar cell carcinomas, and the presence of obscuring factors and artifacts.

# Cytology of Normal Pancreas

Acinar cells predominate in samples of the normal pancreas (Table 1-3). They appear as variably-sized cohesive groups of cells, sometimes with an identifiable central lumen (Figures 1-3, 1-4, 1-5, and 1-6). Single cells are not infrequent. Individual cells are pyramidal or triangular with abundant granular cytoplasm, round, eccentric or central nuclei, and fine granular chromatin. Distinct nucleoli can often be seen.

Ductal cells appear as two-dimensional sheets of cells with a "honeycomb" architecture (Figures 1-7 and 1-8). When

TABLE 1-3. Cytology of the normal pancreas.

Acinar Cells
    Predominant cell type
    Arranged in small to medium-sized cohesive groups; some with lumens
    Variable numbers of single cells
    Pyramidal or triangular shape
    Abundant granular cytoplasm
    Round, eccentric, or central nuclei
    Fine chromatin
    Often distinct nucleoli
Ductal Cells
    Less numerous than acinar cells
    Two-dimensional flat sheets with "honeycomb" appearance
    "Picket-fence" arrangement with basally located nuclei
    Cubodial or columnar shape
    Scant, pale cytoplasm
    Bland-appearing nuclei
    Occasional goblet cells
Islet cells
    Rarely identified in aspirates of normal pancreas

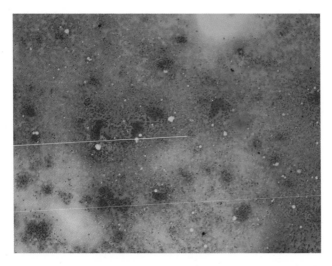

FIGURE 1-3. Aspirate from normal pancreas contains predominantly acinar cells that appear as small cohesive groups of cells and single individual cells. Diff-Quik stain; original magnification, ×20.

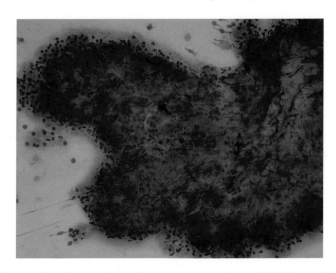

FIGURE 1-4. Large tissue fragments containing individual acini embedded in stroma are commonly aspirated from normal pancreas. Diff-Quik stain; original magnification, ×100.

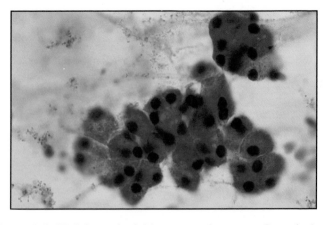

FIGURE 1-5. Well-formed acini from normal pancreas. Papanicolaou stain; original magnification, ×400.

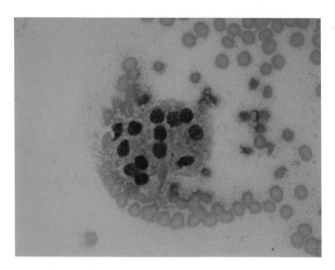

FIGURE 1-6. Individual acinar cells are pyramidal or triangular with abundant granular cytoplasm, round, eccentric or central nuclei, and fine granular chromatin. Distinct nucleoli can often be seen. Diff-Quik stain; original magnification, ×400.

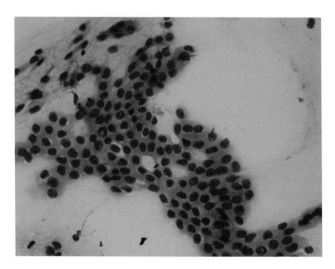

FIGURE 1-7. Normal pancreatic ductal cells arranged in two-dimensional flat sheets with orderly "honeycomb" arrangement. Diff-Quik stain; original magnification, ×100.

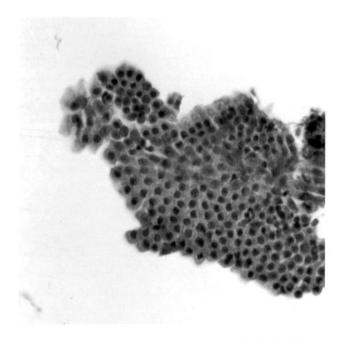

FIGURE 1-8. Normal pancreatic ductal cells. Individual cells appear bland with scant cytoplasm and small, round-to-oval nuclei. Papanicolaou stain; original magnification, ×100.

seen on edge, the ductal cells can have a "picket-fence" appearance with basally located nuclei (Figure 1-9). Individual cells appear bland with scant cytoplasm and small, round-to-oval nuclei. The presence of both acinar and ductal cells usually suggests a benign process. Islet cells are seldom identified in the aspirates of normal pancreas and are characterized by loosely cohesive clusters of bland, round-to-oval cells with central or eccentric round nuclei and granular chromatin.

## Contaminants

Other cell types, for example, mesothelial cells, hepatocytes, and gastrointestinal epithelium or even stromal tissues, may be present in pancreatic FNA (Table 1-4). When

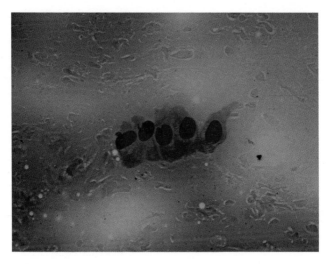

FIGURE 1-9. Normal pancreatic ductal cells arranged in a "picket fence" with basally located nuclei. Diff-Quik stain; original magnification, ×400.

evaluating pancreatic FNA, it is important that pathologists have knowledge of how the specimens are obtained as the cell types of contaminants encountered varies with different approaches.

For example, mesothelial cells and hepatocytes occur more frequently in samples obtained by a percutaneous approach. Mesothelial cells appear as two-dimensional flat sheets of cells with round-to-oval nuclei, a moderate amount of pale cytoplasm, and intercellular windows (Figure 1-10). Normal hepatocytes are polygonal cells with abundant well-defined, granular cytoplasm, round-to-oval nuclei, and prominent nucleoli. (Figure 1-11) Cytoplasmic pigments such as bile and iron may be present.

Despite the use of a stylet while puncturing the gastric or small intestinal wall during EUS-FNA, contamination with gastric or small intestinal tissue still often occurs. It is important to recognize normal gastrointestinal epithelium and stroma to avoid potential diagnostic pitfalls. The epithelium

TABLE 1-4. Possible contaminants of pancreatic FNA.

| Cell types | Approach | Cytologic features |
|---|---|---|
| Mesothelial cells | Percutaneous | Two-dimensional flat sheets<br>Round-to-oval nuclei<br>Moderate amount of pale cytoplasm<br>Intercellular windows |
| Hepatocytes | Percutaneous | Polygonal cells<br>Abundant well-defined, granular cytoplasm<br>Round-to-oval nuclei<br>Prominent nucleoli<br>± Cytoplasmic pigments |
| Bowel mucosa | Endoscopic | |
| Duodenal mucosa | Transduodenal (for lesions in the pancreatic head and ucinate) | Two-dimensional flat sheets with orderly "honeycomb" arrangement<br>Variable number of single cells<br>Round, evenly spaced, and bland-appearing nuclei<br>Pale cytoplasm with well-defined borders<br>Intermixed goblet cells<br>Frequently admixed with thin extracellular mucus |
| Gastric mucosa | Transgastric (for lesions in the pancreatic body and tail) | Two-dimensional flat sheets with orderly "honeycomb" arrangement<br>Variable number of single cells<br>Round, evenly spaced, and bland-appearing nuclei<br>Pale cytoplasm with well-defined borders<br>Goblets cells rare except in intestinal metaplasia<br>Frequently admixed with mucin<br>Parietal cells may be seen |

is characterized by the presence of large and small two-dimensional flat sheets of cells that have an orderly "honeycomb arrangement" with luminal edges at their borders (Figures 1-12 and 1-13). Occasional single cells may be seen. Individual cells have round, evenly spaced, and

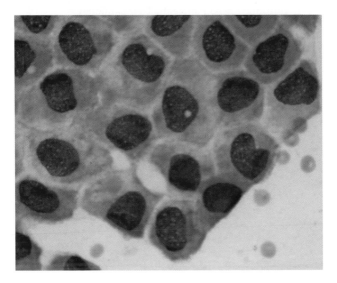

FIGURE 1-10. Mesothelial cells appear as two-dimensional flat sheets with round-to-oval nuclei, a moderate amount of pale cytoplasm, and intercellular windows. Diff-Quik stain; original magnification, ×1000.

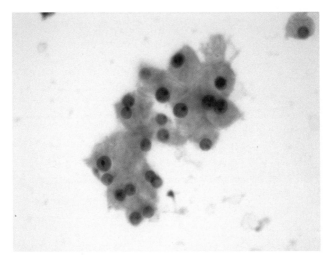

FIGURE 1-11. Normal hepatocytes are polygonal cells with abundant well-defined, granular cytoplasm, cytoplasmic pigments, round-to-oval nuclei, and prominent nucleoli. Papanicolaou stain; original magnification, ×400.

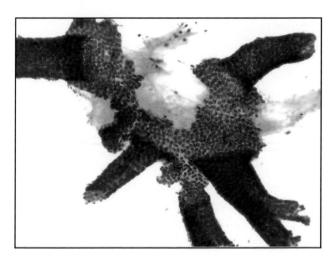

FIGURE 1-12.  Gastric epithelium may be arranged in large fragments with obvious tubular structures. They should not be mistaken as papillary structures because fibrovascular cores are absent. Papanicolaou stain; original magnification, ×20.

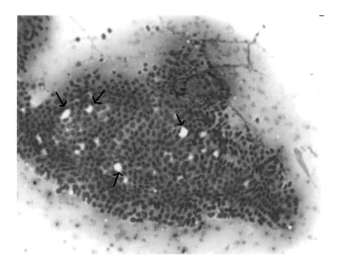

FIGURE 1-13. Duodenal epithelium often forms two-dimensional sheets and has a "starry-sky" appearance because of the goblet cells. Diff-Quik stain; original magnification, ×20.

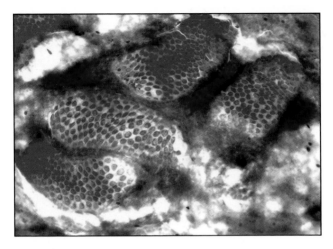

FIGURE 1-14. Gastric and duodenal epithelia have bland cells with round, evenly spaced, nuclei. Diff-Quik stain; original magnification, ×100.

bland-appearing nuclei (Figure 1-14). The cytoplasm is usually pale and has well-defined borders. Goblets cells are frequently seen scattered within duodenal epithelium but rarely within gastric epithelium, except in aspirates from patients with gastric atrophy (Figures 1-15 and 1-16). Because of a lack of goblet cells, gastric foveolar type epithelium may be difficult to distinguish from pancreatic ductal epithelium. The presence of parietal cells nearby would favor a gastric origin (Figure 1-17). Parietal cells, sometimes seen in proximity with gastric foveolar type epithelium, vary in shape from pyramidal to round and have abundant granular cytoplasm, coarse chromatin, and prominent nucleoli. Cells of Brunner glands can sometimes be seen with duodenal epithelium and appear columnar with basally located nuclei and abundant foamy cytoplasm (Figure 1-18). Extracellular mucus may be noted admixed with both duodenal and gastric mucosa and usually appears thin; its distinction from the protenianeous fluid of certain benign pancreatic cysts, such as microcystic adenoma, can be difficult.

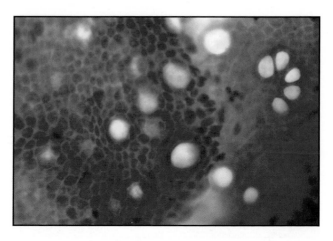

FIGURE 1-15. High magnification of duodenal epithelium with numerous goblet cells. Diff-Quik stain; original magnification, ×200.

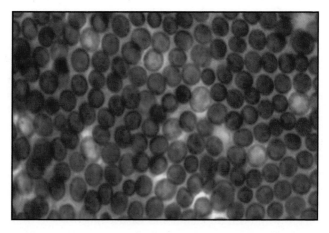

FIGURE 1-16. Duodenal epithelium with scattered goblet cells seen as pale nuclei through the overlying mucin. Papanicolaou stain; original magnification, ×400.

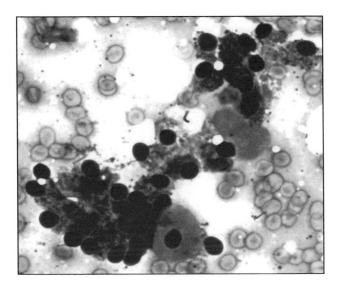

FIGURE 1-17. Parietal cells are pyramidal or round and have abundant granular cytoplasm. Diff-Quik stain; original magnification, ×400.

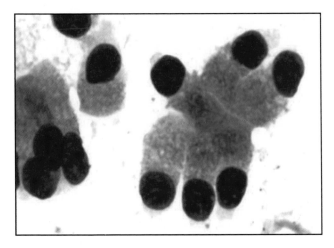

FIGURE 1-18. Cells of Brunner glands are columnar and have basally located nuclei with abundant foamy cytoplasm; in contrast, pancreatic ductal cells tends to have nondescript cytoplasm. Diff-Quik stain; original magnification, ×400.

# Suggested Reading

Brandt KR, Charboneau JW, Stephens DH, Welch TJ, Goellner JR. CT- and US-guided biopsy of the pancreas. Radiology 1993; 187:99–104.

Brugge WR. Pancreatic fine needle aspiration: to do or not to do? J Pancreas 2004;5:282–288.

Centeno BA. Fine needle aspiration biopsy of the pancreas. Clin Lab Med 1998;18:401–427.

David O, Green L, Reddy V, et al. Pancreatic masses: a multi-institutional study of 364 fine-needle aspiration biopsies with histopathologic correlation. Diagn Cytopathol 1998;19:423–427.

de Luna R, Eloubeidi MA, Sheffield MV, et al. Comparison of ThinPrep and conventional preparations in pancreatic fine-needle aspiration biopsy. Diagn Cytopathol 2004;30:71–76.

Di Stasi M, Lencioni R, Solmi L, et al. Ultrasound-guided fine needle biopsy of pancreatic masses: results of a multicenter study. Am J Gastroenterol 1998;93:1329–1333.

Dorge H, Schoendube FA, Schoberer M, Stellbrink C, Voss M, Messmer BJ. Intraoperative amiodarone as prophylaxis against atrial fibrillation after coronary operations. Ann Thorac Surg 2000;69:1358–1362.

Eloubeidi MA, Jhala D, Chhieng DC, et al. Yield of endoscopic ultrasound-guided fine-needle aspiration biopsy in patients with suspected pancreatic carcinoma. Cancer 2003;99:285–292.

Hammel P, Levy P, Voitot H, et al. Preoperative cyst fluid analysis is useful for the differential diagnosis of cystic lesions of the pancreas. Gastroenterology 1995;108:1230–1235.

Henke AC, Jensen CS, Cohen MB. Cytologic diagnosis of adenocarcinoma in biliary and pancreatic duct brushings. Adv Anat Pathol 2002;9:301–308.

Hughes JH, Cohen MB. Fine-needle aspiration of the pancreas. Pathology 1996;4:389–407.

Jhala NC, Jhala DN, Chhieng DC, Eloubeidi MA, Eltoum IA. Endoscopic ultrasound-guided fine-needle aspiration. A cytopathologist's perspective. Am J Clin Pathol 2003;120:351–367.

Lewandrowski K, Lee J, Southern J, Centeno B, Warshaw A. Cyst fluid analysis in the differential diagnosis of pancreatic cysts: a new approach to the preoperative assessment of pancreatic cystic lesions. AJR Am J Roentgenol 1995; 164:815–819.

Nagle JA, Wilbur DC, Pitman MB. Cytomorphology of gastric and duodenal epithelium and reactivity to B72.3: a baseline for comparison to pancreatic lesions aspirated by EUS-FNAB. Diagn Cytopathol 2005;33:381–386.

Voss M, Hammel P, Molas G, et al. Value of endoscopic ultrasound guided fine needle aspiration biopsy in the diagnosis of solid pancreatic masses. Gut 2000;46:244–249.

# 2
# Pancreatic Cytopathology: A Pragmatic Approach

This chapter discusses a general approach for the diagnosis of pancreatic lesions using cytologic samples. An algorithm is supplied that represents the authors' best attempt to recapitulate our own thoughts when we approach samples from the pancreas. Although most cytologists likely use similar processes as they tackle specimens from all parts of the body, an algorithm is destined to be imperfect as it simplifies the multitude of clues that are used to arrive at final diagnoses while also complicating the process by not incorporating the numerous shortcuts that help us to avoid pitfalls. The approach described below utilizes our experience in evaluating pancreatic lesions and is an attempt to put into words a systematic method for the correct identification of most pancreatic lesions by combining clinical, radiographic, and cytologic findings. Specific pitfalls are discussed in the following chapters that describe the individual lesions in more detail.

The World Health Organization has recently systematically reclassified pancreatic neoplasia (Table 2-1). Any cytologist who interprets pancreatic cytologic specimens should have a good understanding of the histopathology of this classification system and should also have a general idea as to the relative frequencies of the various neoplasms as well as their clinical and radiographic or sonographic features.

TABLE 2-1. WHO classification of primary tumors of the exocrine and endocrine pancreas.

Acinar Cell Carcinoma[1]
Ductal Adenocarcinoma[2]
Intraductal Papillary Mucinous Neoplasm[3]
Mucinous Cystic Neoplasm[3]
Pancreatic Endocrine Tumor[4]
Pancreatoblastoma
Serous Cystadenoma[5]
Solid Pseudopapillary Neoplasm[6]

[1]  *Acinar cell carcinomas* can sometimes show mixed differentiation and may show areas of endocrine or ductal differentiation. Such differentiation cannot usually be detected at the time of fine needle aspiration.

[2]  *Ductal Adenocarcinoma* category includes many variants, for example, mucinous noncystic, signet ring cell, adenosquamous, and undifferentiated carcinoma.

[3]  *Intraductal papillary mucinous neoplasms and mucinous cystic neoplasms* are graded depending on the degree of intraepithelial atypia and may both be noninvasive or invasive.

[4]  The WHO classifies *pancreatic endocrine tumors* according to their secretory peptides. Such information is often not available at the time of fine needle aspiration.

[5]  *Serous neoplasms* of the pancreas are almost always benign, although rare cases of malignant serous neoplasms have been reported.

[6]  *Solid pseudopapillary neoplasms* are generally considered to be "borderline" neoplasms. Cases with known metastases are considered to be malignant.

# Clinical and Imaging Data

It is essential for cytologists to know the basic clinical and imaging data for a case before an interpretation is attempted. Onsite interpretation of fine needle aspiration (FNA) specimens, while increasing the diagnostic yield, also allows for direct communication between clinicians and pathologists and the accurate relaying of clinical and radiologic findings. If onsite interpretation is not feasible, the cytologist should make every attempt to acquire this information. A phone call to the individual who collected the specimen often proves informative.

Determining whether a lesion appears solid or cystic represents the starting point for the evaluation of pancreatic

FNA because the differential diagnoses for solid and cystic lesions are quite different. Other data that can be helpful include the age and sex of the patient, the location of the lesion within the pancreas (head, body, or tail), and other radiographic characteristics of the lesion. Some lesions can present with classic clinical and radiographic or sonograpic findings that can be quite helpful (Table 2-2).

## General Interpretation

Figure 2-1(a,b) shows a general algorithm for the inter-pretation of pancreatic cytology samples. As stated above, one begins with knowing whether the lesion appeared solid or cystic by imaging. Most solid or mass lesions will be neoplasms and the cytologist primarily must distinguish pan-creatic ductal adenocarcinomas (PDAs) from benign, non-neoplastic lesions or other less common types of pancreatic neoplasia. With cystic lesions, the pathologist's challenge is to separate mucinous neoplasia or, rarely, cystic examples of typically solid neoplasms such as cystic pancreatic endocrine tumors (PETs), from benign non-neoplastic lesions or serous cysts. Following are some general principles regarding the interpretation and reporting of pancreatic cytology speci-mens. Clinical and cytologic features of the individual lesion will be discussed in depth in the following chapters.

### Solid/Mass Lesions

Most solid or mass lesions of the pancreas are neoplastic and treated, when possible, by resection. Because of this, resection may sometimes be performed without cytologic sampling of the lesions. More recently, endoscopic ultrasound (EUS) has come to be increasingly used for the identification, assessment, and staging of pancreatic neoplasia. In addition, EUS enables tissue sampling by FNA and, as a result, lesions are often biopsied prior to surgery. Subsequent man-agement decisions are often made after imaging and FNA.

TABLE 2-2. Clinical and imaging features of primary pancreatic neoplasms.

| Neoplasm | Clinical features | | | Imaging features | |
| --- | --- | --- | --- | --- | --- |
| | Symptoms and Signs | Age | Gender | Character | Location |
| Acinar cell carcinoma | Enzymatic release (uncommon) | >50 years old | M > W | Solid, somewhat circumscribed | Head |
| Ductal adenocarcinoma | Painless jaundice | >50 years old | M > W | Infiltrating; CBD or pancreatic duct obstruction | Head |
| Intraductal papillary mucinous neoplasm | Chronic pancreatitis | >50 years old | M > W | Cystic appearing with communication with the ductal system; main duct dilatation; papillary excrescences | Head |
| Mucinous cystic neoplasm | Incidental; nonspecific symptoms | Adult | W | Multilocular cystic lesion; no ductal communication | Body or tail |
| Pancreatic endocrine tumor | Syndrome secondary to peptide hormone production, e.g., hypoglycemia | Adult | M = W | Solid, circumscribed mass | Tail |
| Pancreatoblastoma | Nonspecific symptoms | <10 years old | M = W | Solid mass with pushing borders | Head |
| Serous cystadenoma | Nonspecific symptoms | Adult | W > M | Multiple small cysts with central scar | Body and tail |
| Solid pseudopapillary neoplasm | Nonspecific symptoms | Young and middle aged | W | Solid and cystic lesion; calcified | Tail |

Figure 2-1. (a) Algorithm for the interpretation of pancreatic cytologic samples, part 1.

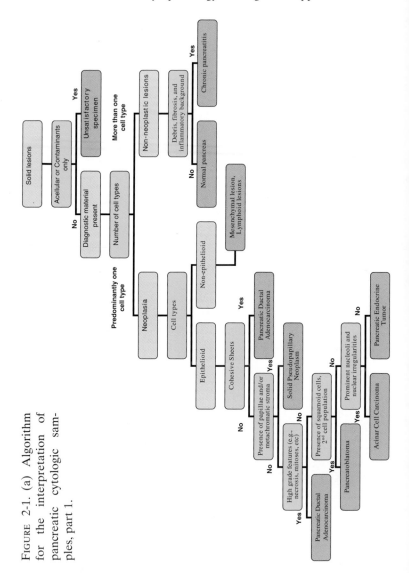

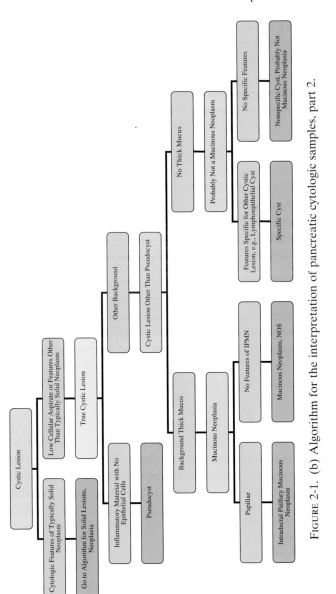

FIGURE 2-1. (b) Algorithm for the interpretation of pancreatic cytologic samples, part 2.

Information from FNA is often helpful and necessary when patients are deemed not to be surgical candidates.

Samples from solid or mass lesions should first be assessed for cellularity. The pathologist must then distinguish normal tissues from lesional tissues. Often this necessitates distinguishing contaminants from lesional tissue. This is especially true with bile duct brushings and samples obtained by endoscopic ultrasound-fine needle aspiration (EUS-FNA). With bile duct brushing, biliary epithelium, which may show severely reactive changes secondary to either stent placement or lithiasis, must be recognized as different from neoplasia. Samples obtained by EUS-FNA often contain abundant gastric or duodenal epithelium that also must be distinguished from pathologic material. Finally, pathologists must also be able to recognize normal pancreatic parenchyma and not confuse it with less common types of pancreatic neoplasia such as acinar cell carcinoma.

Once tissue is recognized as abnormal, non-neoplastic disease, most commonly chronic pancreatitis, must then be distinguished from neoplasia. Clinical and imaging findings may be similar for both chronic pancreatitis and neoplasia, especially PDA. Furthermore, some degree of chronic pancreatitis typically accompanies most pancreatic neoplasia and may be sampled at the same time as the neoplastic tissue.

The distinction between the various types of pancreatic neoplasia is not always necessary, but is often straightforward, as most neoplasms will represent PDA, which does not share many overlapping cytologic features with other types of pancreatic neoplasia. Some variants of PDA, however, may appear obviously malignant, but can be harder to separate from other tumors. In such cases, immunocytochemistry may be helpful.

With other pancreatic neoplasms, cytologic features alone may not always allow for a definitive diagnosis. The use of immunocytochemistry using a small panel can be helpful in most instances. The combined phenotypic expression with antibodies to pancytokeratin (cocktail), synaptophysin, chromogranin, and vimentin will define most primary pancreatic neoplasms when PDA is excluded by morphology alone (Table 2-3). Acinar cell carcinomas will react with antibodies

TABLE 2-3. Immunochemical reactions of solid pancreatic neoplasms.

| Neoplasm | CK | CD56 | SYN | CHR | VIM | CT | AAT | AACT | LIP | TRP |
|---|---|---|---|---|---|---|---|---|---|---|
| PDA | + | − | − | − | − | − | − | − | − | − |
| PET | + | + | + | + | −* | − | − | − | − | − |
| SPT | −** | + | −** | − | + | + | + | + | − | − |
| ACC | + | − | − | − | − | + | + | + | + | + |

Abbreviations: AACT, alpha-1-antichymotrysin; AAT, alpha-1-antitrypsin; ACC, acinar cell carcinoma; CHR, chromogranin; CK, pancytokeratin; CT, chymotrypsin; LIP, lipase; PDA, pancreatic ductal adenocarcinoma; PET, pancreatic endocrine tumor; SPT, solid pseudopapillary neoplasm; SYN, synaptophysin; TRP, trypsin; VIM, vimentin.
* Up to 20% to 30% of PETs may be immunoreactive for vimentin.
** Occasional focal immunoreactivity for CK and SYN has been noted in SPTs. Rare SPTs may show diffuse, weak reactivity for SYN.

to cytokeratins, but should not generally react with antibodies to vimentin or endocrine antigens. Although antibodies to acinar cell enzymes can also be helpful, most laboratories will not carry these markers due to the relative infrequency of these tumors and their limited use outside of this context. Most PETs will react with antibodies to cytokeratins and endocrine antigens and will not react with antibodies to vimentin. Finally, solid pseudopapillary neoplasms should react with antibodies to vimentin and will only show limited reactivity with antibodies to cytokeratins or synaptophysin and chromogranin. They may show more diffuse reactivity with antibodies to less specific endocrine antigens, such as CD56 or NSE and to some acinar cell antigens.

## Cystic Lesions

Most pancreatic cysts are pseudocysts and are often associated with other diseases of the pancreas (Table 2-4). Patients with pseudocysts often have known histories of pancreatitis secondary to alcoholism or biliary lithiasis. Cystic neoplasms, however, have been increasingly identified because of the increased use of radiographic imaging. Importantly, many of these have nonspecific imaging characteristics and the differential diagnosis frequently includes mucinous cystic neoplasms and intraductal papillary mucinous neoplasms. As current surgical dogma indicates that such lesions should often be resected because of increased risk for either concurrent or subsequent development of invasive adenocarcinoma, cytopathologists are often called to identify these challenging lesions.

Most current studies that have retrospectively evaluated the cytologic features of mucinous neoplasms of the pancreas have touted the importance of the identification of thick mucus and atypical mucinous epithelia. Undoubtedly, in the right clinical context, finding thick mucus in these samples in air-dried, Diff-Quik preparations is very predictive of pancreatic mucinous neoplasia. However, the importance of the finding mucus alone and how much such a finding contributes to the diagnosis of any particular case is not known. Furthermore, in studies evaluating the identification of mucus prospectively with pancreatic cytology samples, other markers, such as cyst fluid CEA levels, appear to be more sensitive for the identification of pancreatic mucinous neoplasia (Table 2-5).

TABLE 2-4. Pancreatic cysts.

Non-neoplastic
  Inflammatory
    Pseudocyst
    Infectious
  Congenital
  Other
Neoplastic
  Mucinous
    Mucinous cystic neoplasm
    Intraductal papillary mucinous neoplasm
  Serous
    Serous cystadenoma
  Other
    Acinar cell cystadenoma
    Lymphoepithelial cyst
    Other typically solid neoplasms

TABLE 2-5. Chemical analysis of pancreatic cyst fluid.

| Cutoff | Diagnosis* |
|--------|-----------|
| Amylase < 250 U/L | Serous cystadenoma and mucinous neoplasm |
| CEA < 5 ng/mL | Serous cystadenoma and pseudocyst |
| CEA > 800 ng/mL | Mucinous neoplasm |
| CA 19-9 < 36 U/mL | Serous cystadenoma and pseudocyst |

* High specificity and positive predictive value.
*Source*: Modified from van der Waaij LA, van Dullemen HM, Porte RJ. Cyst fluid analysis in the differential diagnosis of pancreatic cystic lesions: a pooled analysis. Gastrointest Endosc 2005;62:383–389.

## Reporting

The diagnostic reporting of anatomic specimens is critical to the clinical management of the patient. Although cytologists are generally expected to offer a specific diagnosis for all samples, such specificity is not always possible and/or necessary. This is especially true for cytologic specimens with which the pathologist's primary role is often to provide information that will guide proper triaging of the patient.

Currently, there are no published criteria for the assessment of adequacy with pancreatic cytology specimens. Adequacy is thus defined by the pathologist on a case-to-case basis and is dependent on various factors, including the operator, the method of collection, and the characteristics of the particular pancreatic lesion sampled.

With solid lesions, the most common clinical and imaging mimic of a neoplasm is chronic pancreatitis. Unfortunately, some degree of chronic pancreatitis is almost always present with any given neoplasm. Radiologists and sonographers are sometimes not able to identify one from the other and, furthermore, cannot necessarily tell where one lesion ends and the other begins. Thus, in the face of a mass lesion, it is currently unclear what the predictive value of the cytologic diagnosis of chronic pancreatitis is. Even if no atypical ductal cells are seen, a significant portion (approximately 10%–20%) of such cases turn out to be PDAs.

How many ductal cells with malignant features are necessary for the diagnosis of PDA? This question also has not been answered. The cellularity of pancreatic specimens varies greatly and, except for severe acute pancreatitis, which is rarely sampled, there is little overlap between the morphologic features of PDA and other disease, especially with samples gathered by FNA. The one obvious mimic is high-grade pancreatic intraepithelial neoplasia, which may be seen in cases of chronic pancreatitis and is more likely to be encountered with older patients. Many who have much experience with pancreatic FNAs have encountered the rare false-positive cases, for which cytologic samplings have been diagnostic of PDA while the resected specimens are free of invasive tumor yet contain high-grade pancreatic intraepithelial neoplasia. Although no actual numbers are published regarding this, our anecdotal experience suggests that this is extremely uncommon (i.e., less than 1% of aspirates diagnosed as PDA). On the other hand, low cellularity samples from actual invasive PDAs appear to be much more common and thus "backing off" with one's diagnosis due to low cellularity may not be warranted. Unlike bile duct brushings, samples from pancreatic FNA interpreted as "suspicious" or even "atypical" are almost always found to be PDA at resection. That said, prudence is recommended, particularly if the clinical and/or radiologic findings are not consistent with the cytologic interpretation of malignancy.

Although solid lesions can usually be diagnosed definitively, samples from cystic lesions may often require more "descriptive diagnoses" (Figure 2-2). If the specimen is cellular, definitive diagnoses can usually be made. However, it should be noted that the diagnosis of "adenocarcinoma" for cellular cystic lesions does not necessarily imply an invasive process. Both mucinous cystic neoplasms and intraductal papillary mucinous neoplasms can show intraepithelial lesions that are indistinguishable from invasive adenocarcinomas by cytology sampling alone (i.e., adenocarcinoma in situ).

In many instances, aspirates from cystic lesions are hypocellular and the rare epithelial cells may appear bland and indistinguishable from gastrointestinal contaminant. In such cases, descriptive diagnoses with the mentioning of the presence or absence of thick, extracellular mucus may be

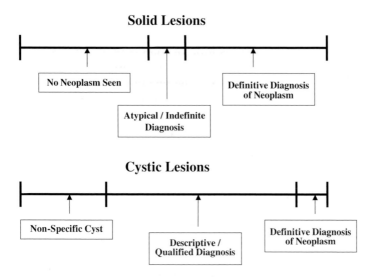

FIGURE 2-2. Reporting of cytologic samples from solid versus cystic pancreatic lesions.

helpful. The positive and negative predictive values of such findings are not known.

The use of a multitiered system for the general categorization of cytologic samples from various sites has some advantages, including the standardization of a particular laboratory's reports. Furthermore, such standardization may help clinicians interpret the reports. Table 2-6 lists the reporting terminology of a five-tiered system that many use. A negative or inadequate diagnosis in the presence of a clinical and/or

TABLE 2-6.  Reporting terminology.

Negative for malignancy
Atypical cells present
Suspicious for malignancy
Positive for malignancy
Unsatisfactory

radiological suspicious lesion may signify sampling error, requiring further evaluation. An atypical diagnosis is reserved for aspirates showing cytologic atypia that exceeds that of reactive/reparative process but is not diagnostic of a malignancy. A suspicious diagnosis is used for specimens that demonstrate most but not all features of malignancy, that is, features that are quantitatively or qualitatively insufficient for a definitive diagnosis of malignancy. For the four satisfactory categories, a specific diagnosis or a differential diagnosis should be rendered if possible.

One needs to be aware that a multitiered reporting system may be difficult to apply to certain pancreatic lesions such as cystic neoplasms. The latter are morphologically heterogeneous and are often impossible to diagnose definitively prospectively. As a result, "atypical" diagnoses will be made frequently with a description of the cytologic finding and a list of plausible differential diagnoses.

# 3
# Pancreatic Ductal Adenocarcinoma and Its Variants

Pancreatic ductal adenocarcinoma (PDA) and its variants comprise 85% to 90% of all pancreatic cancers. It is usually a disease of older individuals and affected patients are often in their seventh to eighth decades of life. The disease is uncommon in patients 40 years or younger and men are affected slightly more frequently than women. The classic clinical symptomatic triad includes epigastric pain with radiation to the back, jaundice, and weight loss. Unfortunately, these findings are nonspecific and can occur in patients with other malignancies or benign diseases, such as gallstones. In addition, many patients only have minimal or vague symptoms when the disease is still curable and in the early stage, especially when it arises in the body or tail of the pancreas.

Over half of the PDAs arise in the pancreatic head, 15% in the body, and 5% in the tail. Up to 20% of PDAs present with multiple foci of tumor throughout the pancreas. Tumors usually appear hypodense by contrast-enhanced computed tomography. Endoscopic ultrasound (EUS) generally reveals a heterogeneous solid mass with irregular and hypoechoic borders. Similar changes by either imaging technique, however, can be seen in patients with other pancreatic tumors and chronic pancreatitis. Imaging can provide information about the local extent of the tumor, the involvement of regional vascular structures, and the presence of nodal or hepatic metastases.

TABLE 3-1. Approach to diagnosing pancreatic ductal carcinoma.

Low power
   Cellularity
   Cellular arrangement
   Cohesiveness
   Background
Intermediate power
   Composition of cell groups
   Organization of cell groups—loss or maintenance of polarity, degree of
     nuclear crowding/overlapping, and two- versus three-dimensionality
High power
   Nuclear features—nuclear size, nuclear contours, nuclear-to-cytoplasmic
     ratio, chromatin pattern, degree of anisonucleosis, presence or absence
     of nucleoli, mitotic activity, etc.

# General Diagnostic Approach

Most cases of PDA present as solid masses and are sampled to exclude other disease processes. As PDA is the most common cytologic neoplastic diagnosis made with samples from the pancreas, a consistent approach to this diagnosis is prudent (Table 3-1). One should begin by examining the specimen at low power to assess the cellularity, the cellular arrangement, the degree of cohesiveness, and the background. Examination at intermediate power provides information about the composition and organization of the cell groups, such as degree of nuclear crowding and polarity. Finally, nuclear features such as nuclear contours, chromatin pattern, nuclear size, nuclear to cytoplasmic ratios, degree of anisonucleosis, and mitotic activity, are best evaluated at high power. By attending to all these features systematically, one can minimize the risk of misinterpretation due to over-reliance on any single feature.

# Diagnostic Criteria

Typically, aspirates of PDA are highly cellular. The background can be clean, inflammatory, mucinous, or necrotic (Figures 3-1 and 3-2). Ductal cells predominate, usually in the

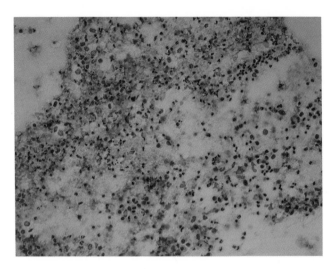

FIGURE 3-1. Pancreatic ductal adenocarcinoma with an extensive inflammatory background. Such a tumor can be confused with chronic pancreatitis. Diff-Quik stain; original magnification, ×20.

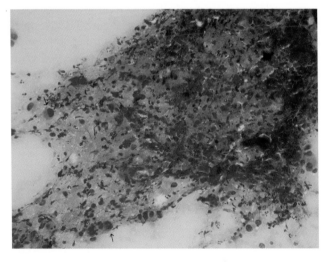

FIGURE 3-2. Pancreatic ductal adenocarcinoma with a necrotic background. Arrows indicate the presence of scattered malignant cells admixed with necrotic debris. Diff-Quik stain; original magnification, ×20.

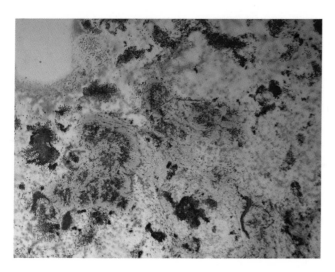

FIGURE 3-3. Aspirates of pancreatic ductal adenocarcinomas are often highly cellular. Neoplastic ductal cells form sheets, clusters, and three-dimensional aggregates. Diff-Quik stain; ×20.

absence of other cellular components (Figure 3-3). Neoplastic ductal cells are arranged in groups and form sheets, clusters, and three-dimensional aggregates. Within these cell groups, the cells are often overcrowded and arranged in a haphazard fashion (Figure 3-4). Variable numbers of isolated, atypical cells are also often identified. Some degree of nuclear pleomorphism and atypia are often present but can be quite subtle in cases of well-differentiated adenocarcinoma. Table 3-2 summarizes the cytologic findings of PDA.

## Well-Differentiated Adenocarcinoma

A low power clue for the diagnosis of well-differentiated PDA is the finding of numerous large sheets of ductal cells in the absence of acinar or islet cells. At a quick glance, the sheets appear two-dimensional with a "honeycomb"

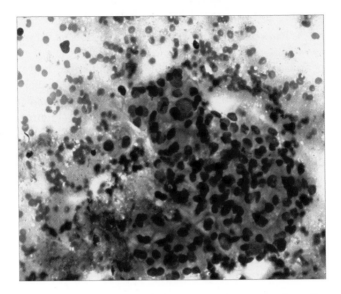

FIGURE 3-4. Within the neoplastic ductal cell groups, the cells are often overcrowded and arranged in a haphazard fashion. Diff-Quik stain; original magnification, ×100.

TABLE 3-2. Cytologic features of pancreatic ductal carcinoma.

**General**
  High cellularity
  Background: clean, inflammatory, mucinous, and necrotic
  Predominantly ductal cells
  Cell groups with overcrowding and/or disorderly arrangement
  Isolated atypical cells
  Nuclear atypia—ranging from mild to severe
    Nuclear enlargement (at least 2× the size of red blood cells)
    Irregular nuclear contours
    Coarse chromatin
    Macronucleoli
    Bi- and multinucleation
    Mitotic figures
**Well-differentiated ductal adenocarcinoma**
  Numerous large, two-dimensional sheets of ductal cells
  "Drunken honeycomb" appearance—unevenly distributed nuclei within
    the sheets
  Well-defined cytoplasmic borders
  Low nuclear-to-cytoplasmic ratios in some cells
  Scattered, isolated atypical cells
**Moderately and poorly differentiated ductal adenocarcinomas**
  Numerous three-dimensional cell groups and aggregates
  Nuclear crowding and overlapping
  Increased number of single atypical cells
  Increased degree of nuclear atypia
  "Tombstone cells"—very large, very tall, atypical, isolated columnar cells

appearance (Figure 3-5). On closer examination, however, the individual cells appear spread out and the nuclei are unevenly distributed, thus giving the sheets the classically described appearance of "drunken honeycombs" (Figures 3-6 and 3-7). Occasional cells will have abundant cytoplasm and, thus, low nuclear-to-cytoplasmic ratios (Figure 3-8). In addition, individual cells have well-defined cell borders (Figure 3-9). Severely atypical individual cells are often few in numbers; however, their identification can be extremely helpful for making a diagnosis of PDA (Figure 3-10).

Nuclear changes can be subtle. Nuclear enlargement, with nuclei at least twice the size of red blood cells, can be seen with at least some of the neoplastic cells. Irregular nuclear contours with folds, clefts, and grooves, are present in over 90% of cases (Figure 3-11). Other features such as hyperchromasia, coarse chromatin, prominent nucleoli, mitotic figures, and bi- and multinucleation are variably present.

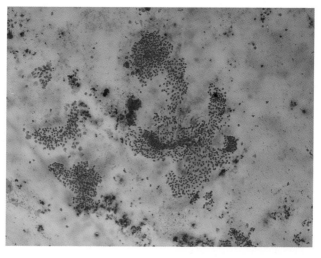

FIGURE 3-5. Well-differentiated pancreatic ductal adenocarcinoma with numerous sheets of ductal cells. Diff-Quik stain; original magnification, ×40.

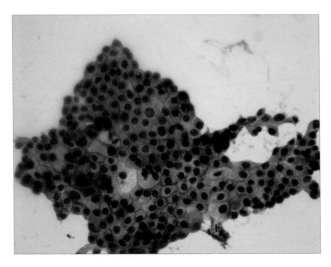

FIGURE 3-6. Well-differentiated pancreatic ductal adenocarcinoma with a two-dimensional sheet showing a somewhat "honeycomb architecture." Papanicolaou stain; original magnification, ×100.

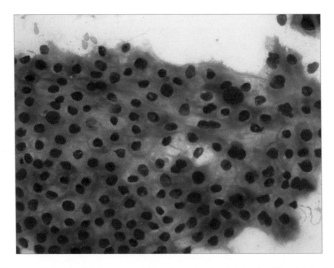

FIGURE 3-7. On higher magnification, the individual cells within the sheet appear spread out and the nuclei are unevenly distributed, thus giving the sheets the classically described appearance of "drunken honeycombs." Diff-Quik stain; original magnification, ×200.

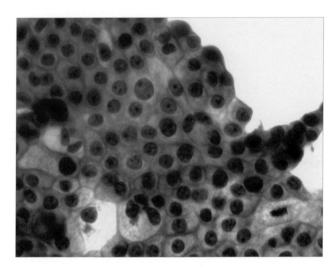

FIGURE 3-8. Not infrequently, the ductal cells of well-differentiated pancreatic ductal adenocarcinoma will have abundant cytoplasm and low nuclear-to-cytoplasmic ratios. Papanicolaous stain; original magnification, ×200.

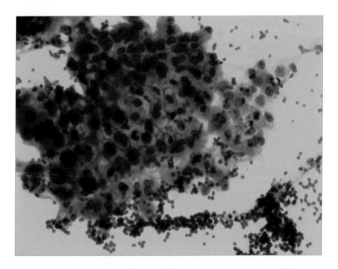

FIGURE 3-9. Individual cells within the sheets have well-defined cell borders. Papanicolaous stain; original magnification, ×200.

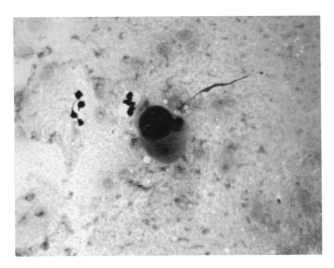

FIGURE 3-10. Scattered large pleomorphic cells with irregular nuclear contours and hyperchromasia are present in the majority of well-differentiated pancreatic ductal adenocarcinomas. Diff-Quik stain; original magnification, ×400.

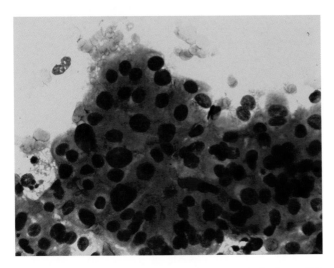

FIGURE 3-11. Individuals neoplastic ductal cells display mild-to-moderate cytologic atypia including nuclear enlargement thus providing ample anisonuculeosis. Diff-Quik stain; original magnification, ×200.

Neoplastic cells have delicate and nondescript cytoplasm. Cytoplasmic vacuoles are quite common. Rare large cytoplasmic vacuoles can be seen and should not be confused with goblet cells seen with small bowel contaminant that may be sampled by endoscopic ultrasound–fine needle aspiration (EUS-FNA).

## Moderately and Poorly Differentiated Adenocarcinoma

The diagnosis of moderately and poorly differentiated adenocarcinomas usually poses little challenge for cytologists. The aspirates are cellular and demonstrate sheets and three-dimensional groups of crowded cells admixed with a variable number of single cells (Figures 3-12, 3-13, 3-14, and 3-15). A noted characteristic feature is the presence of "tombstone cells," which are very large, tall, atypical, single columnar cells (Figures 3-16 and 3-17). This finding is so characteristic

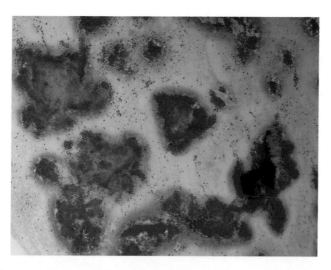

FIGURE 3-12. A cellular aspirate of a moderately differentiated pancreatic ductal adenocarcinoma. Diff-Quik stain; original magnification, ×40.

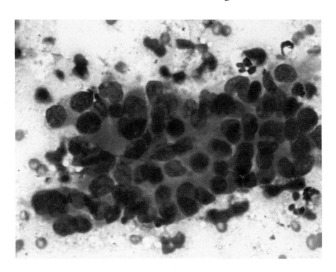

FIGURE 3-13. Intermediate magnification of a moderately differentiated pancreatic ductal adenocarcinoma showing a cluster of ductal cells with nuclear overlap and crowding. Diff-Quik stain; original magnification, ×100.

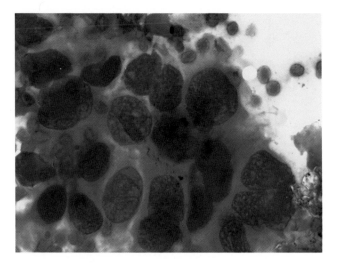

FIGURE 3-14. Individual neoplastic ductal cells from moderately differentiated pancreatic ductal adenocarcinoma display easily discernible nuclear abnormalities, such as nuclear enlargement and coarse chromatin. Diff-Quik stain; original magnification, ×400.

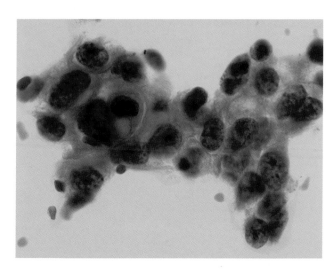

FIGURE 3-15. Prominent macro-nucleoli and irregular nuclear contours are frequently seen in moderately differentiated pancreatic ductal adenocarcinoma. Papanicolaou stain; original magnification, ×400.

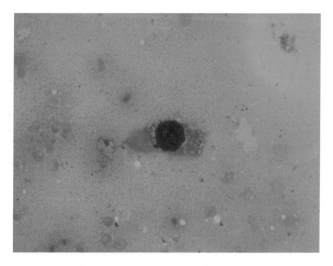

FIGURE 3-16. An example of "tombstone cell": a large, tall, atypical, single columnar cell. Diff-Quik stain; original magnification, ×400.

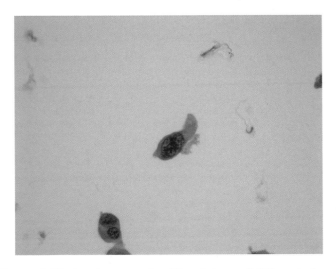

FIGURE 3-17. Another example of "tombstone cell." Papanicolaous stain; original magnification, ×400.

of PDA that when it is noted in aspirates of metastatic adeno-carcinoma, one should think of metastatic PDA.

## Variants of Pancreatic Ductal Carcinoma

Variants of PDA account for about 10% to 15% of all pancreatic malignancies. In general, these tumors demonstrate features typical of epithelial malignancy. The distinction between ordinary PDA and its variants is usually not clinically important because these tumors do not differ significantly in terms of prognosis or management. The exceptions are signet ring cell carcinoma and small cell undifferentiated carcinoma; with only supportive treatment, the prognosis of patients with these tumors is extremely poor with survival in terms of weeks. However, partial and even complete tumor remission has been reported in patients with small cell undifferentiated carcinoma when treated with chemotherapy. Table 3-3 summarizes the cytologic features of some variants of PDA.

TABLE 3-3. Variants of pancreatic ductal carcinomas.

| Variants | Cytologic features | Comments/caveats |
|---|---|---|
| Adenosquamous carcinoma | Presence of both malignant glandular and squamous components | Cells with squamoid features can be seen in conventional pancreatic ductal carcinoma |
| Anaplastic carcinoma | Presence of large, bizarre multinucleated giant cells and/or pleomorphic spindle-shaped cells; phagocytosis of inflammatory cells is frequent | Must exclude other families of tumors, e.g., melanoma, lymphoma, sarcoma, etc. |
| Osteoclastic giant cell tumor | Presence of neoplastic mononucleated spindle-shaped to epithelioid cells and non-neoplastic multinucleated osteoclastic-like giant cells | The presence of bizarre, multinucleated giant cells excludes this diagnosis |
| Signet ring cell carcinoma | Cells with large cytoplasmic vacuoles that push the atypical nuclei to the periphery | Occasional signet ring cells are often associated with conventional pancreatic ductal carcinomas |
| Foamy gland adenocarcinoma | Glands composed of cells with abundant foamy cytoplasm, basally located hyperchromatic nuclei, and an apical brush border-like cytoplasmic condensation | Often associated with conventional pancreatic ductal carcinoma |
| Small cell undifferentiated carcinoma | Small cells ($2\times$–$4\times$ the size of a small lymphocyte) with scant cytoplasm, "salt and pepper" chromatin, and indistinct nucleoli; nuclear molding is often apparent | Metastatic small cell carcinoma to the pancreas needs to be excluded |

## Adenosquamous Carcinoma

This variant accounts for less than 5% of all PDA and is characterized by the presence of malignant glandular and squamous components; by definition, the squamous component should account for at least 30% of the tumor on tissue sections of the resected malignancy. Because adenoaquamous carcinomas are usually high grade, recognition of their malignant nature is usually straightforward with cytologic samples. Distinguishing the tumors from ordinary PDAs requires the identification of both malignant glandular and squamous cells. The presence of malignant keratinized squamous cells is the most reliable evidence of squamous differentiation (Figures 3-18, 3-19, and 3-20). This feature, however, may be focal and easily overlooked. Furthermore, neoplastic cells of conventional PDAs can also demonstrate some squamoid features, such as dense cytoplasm and well-defined cell borders (Figures 3-21 and 3-22). It is very important that

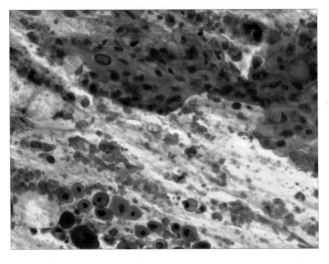

FIGURE 3-18. An example of an adenosquamous carcinoma showing both its glandular and squamous components. Papanicolaou stain; original magnification, ×40.

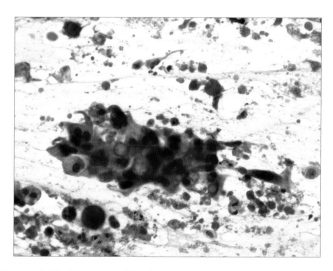

FIGURE 3-19. High magnification of an adenosquamous carcinoma with markedly atypical keratinized squamous cells. Vacuolated glandular cells are also noted. Papanicolaou stain; original magnification, ×200.

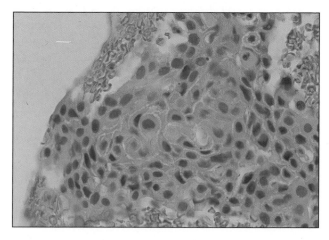

FIGURE 3-20. Cell block preparation showing the malignant squamous component of an adenosquamous carcinoma. Hemotoxylin and eosin stain; original magnification, ×200.

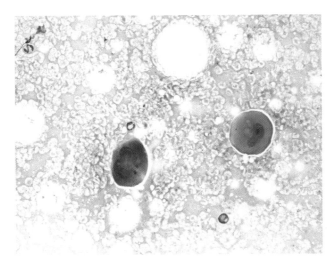

FIGURE 3-21. Neoplastic ductal cells with squamoid features such as dense cytoplasm and well-defined cell borders can be seen in conventional pancreatic ductal adenocarcinomas. Diff-Quik stain; original magnification, ×400.

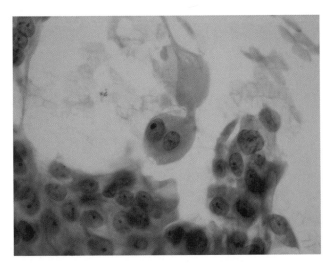

FIGURE 3-22. Another example of neoplastic squamoid ductal cells. Papanicolaou stain; original magnification, ×400.

cytopathologists know of this variant and of the propensity of pancreatic PDAs to show squamous differentiation so as to not confuse these with metastases to the pancreas.

Anaplastic Carcinoma

Aspirates from these uncommon tumors are characterized by the presence of large, bizarre, multinucleated giant cells and/ or pleomorphic spindle-shaped cells. The tumors have also been referred to as "pleomorphic giant cell carcinomas" (Figure 3-23) and "sarcomatoid carcinomas" (Figures 3-24, and 3-25), depending on their dominant morphology. They share similar age and gender distributions with conventional PDAs, but arise more frequently in the pancreatic body and tail. These tumors are obviously malignant cytologically, but ancillary studies may be required to show their epithelial origin. The differential diagnosis for these tumors can include

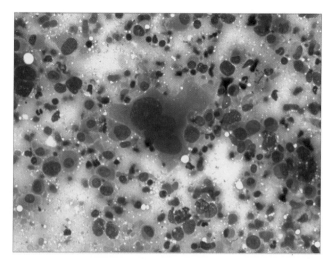

FIGURE 3-23. A pleomorphic giant cell from a case of anaplastic carcinoma. Diff-Quik stain; original magnification, ×400.

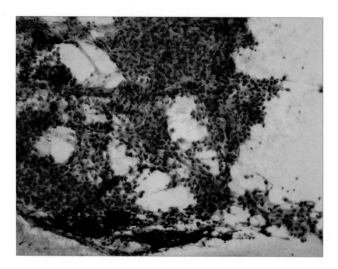

FIGURE 3-24. Low power image showing large tissue fragments consisting predominantly of spindle cells from a sarcomatoid carcinoma. Papanicolaou stain; original magnification, ×40.

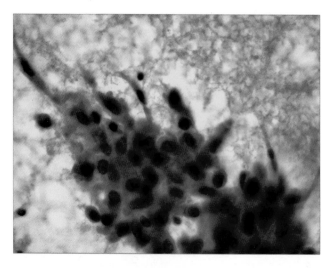

FIGURE 3-25. High power image showing a mixture of atypical spindle and epithelioid cells in a sarcomatoid carcinoma. Papanicolaou stain; original magnification, ×400.

melanoma, sarcoma, lymphoma, and metastasis. Immunocytochemistry with antibodies to cytokeratin may be helpful for
confirming the epithelial nature of these tumors (Figure 3-26).
The absence of the expression of other antigens, such as CD45
or S100, can be helpful for excluding other malignancies.

Osteoclastic Giant Cell Tumor

Aspirates from these tumors are characterized by the
presence of two distinct cell populations: neoplastic mono-
nucleated spindle-shaped to epithelioid cells (Figures 3-27
and 3-28) and non-neoplastic multinucleated osteoclastic-
like giant cells (Figures 3-29 and 3-30). The presence of
bizarre, multinucleated tumor giant cells would exclude this
diagnosis, and, instead, tumors with such cells should be classified as anaplastic carcinomas. Aspirates from inflammatory
or reactive conditions, such as fat necrosis, may also have
benign giant cells and should be considered in the differential
diagnosis. Some have suggested that this tumor may have a
more favorable prognosis than conventional PDA.

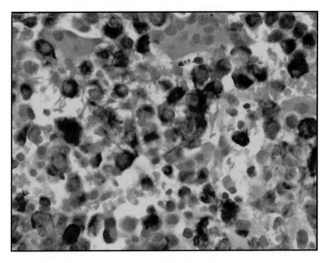

Figure 3-26. Immunoreactivity for cytokeratin confirms the epithelial nature of this anaplastic carcinoma. Cell block; original magnification, ×400.

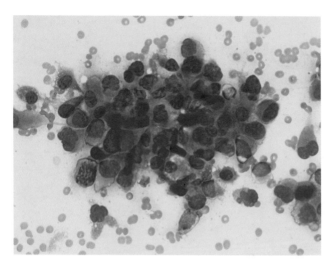

FIGURE 3-27. The mononuclear component of an osteoclastic giant cell variant of pancreatic ductal adenocarcinoma. The mononuclear cells appear either epithelioid or spindle-shaped and demonstrate conspicuous cytologic atypia. Diff-Quik stain; original magnification, ×400.

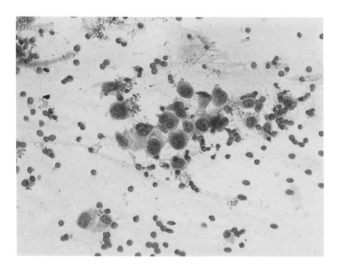

FIGURE 3-28. Another example of the mononuclear neoplastic cells of an osteoclastic giant cell variant of pancreatic ductal adenocarcinoma. Papanicolaou stain; original magnification, ×400.

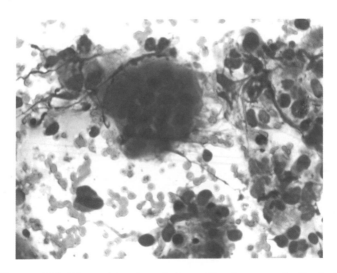

FIGURE 3-29. The multinucleated giant cells of an osteoclastic giant cell variant resemble osteoclasts. In contrast to the mononuclear cells, the nuclei of the multinucleated giant cells lack cytologic aytpia. Diff-Quik stain; original magnification, ×400.

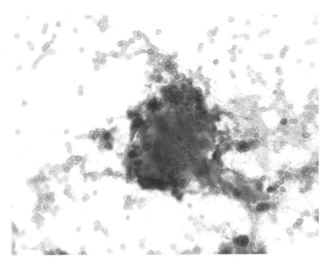

FIGURE 3-30. Another example of multinucleated giant cell in an osteoclastic giant cell variant of pancreatic ductal adenocarcinoma. Papanicolaou stain; original magnification, ×400.

## Signet Ring Cell Carcinoma

It is not uncommon to find occasional signet ring cells in an aspirate from an otherwise typical PDA (Figure 3-31). On the other hand, pure signet ring cell carcinomas of the pancreas are extremely rare and very aggressive malignancies. The cytologic features are identical to those of other gastrointestinal (GI) signet ring carcinomas and the neoplastic cells are predominately single or isolated and contain a large cytoplasmic vacuole that indents an eccentrically located and atypical nucleus (Figure 3-32). The differential diagnosis should include the direct extension of a gastric signet ring cell carcinoma of the stomach into the pancreas.

## Foamy Gland Adenocarcinoma

This is a somewhat newly described histologic pattern of PDA that is characterized by the presence of neoplastic glands lined by cells with abundant clear, finely vacuolated

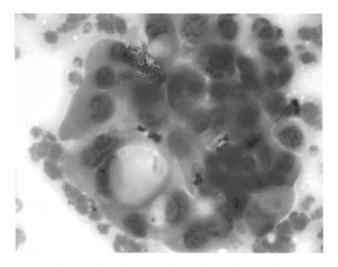

FIGURE 3-31. Occasional signet ring cells can be seen in a conventional pancreatic ductal adenocarcinoma. Diff-Quik stain; original magnification, ×400.

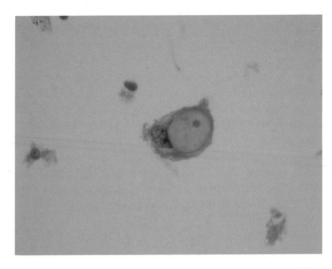

FIGURE 3-32. An example of signet ring cell carcinoma with predominately single/isolated signet ring cells that contain a large cytoplasmic vacuole that indents an eccentricly located and atypical nucleus. Papanicolaou stain; original magnification, ×400.

cytoplasm; basally located, irregular, hyperchromatic nuclei; and a brush border-like zone created by apical cytoplasmic condensation (Figures 3-33, 3-34, and 3-35). Although no clinical or biologic significance is associated with this histologic pattern, it may present a diagnostic challenge because of its relatively bland cytologic appearance. Fortunately, cytologic features of conventional PDA are present almost universally.

## Small Cell Undifferentiated Carcinoma

This rare but highly aggressive malignancy shares similar cytologic morphology with small cell carcinomas from other sites, such as the lung (Figures 3-36 and 3-37). Aspirates are usually cellular and consist of small cells (2–4 times the size of small lymphocytes) with scant cytoplasm, granular or "salt-and-pepper" chromatin, and indistinct nucleoli. Nuclear molding is usually apparent. These tumors often show

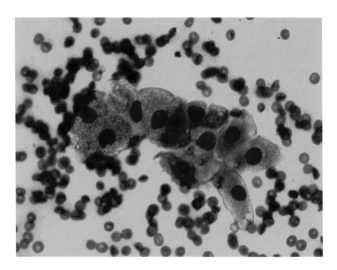

FIGURE 3-33. An example of the foamy gland variant of pancreatic ductal adenocarcinoma that is characterized by neoplastic glands lined by cells with abundant clear, finely vacuolated cytoplasm and basally located, irregular, hyperchromatic nuclei. Diff-Quik stain; original magnification, ×400.

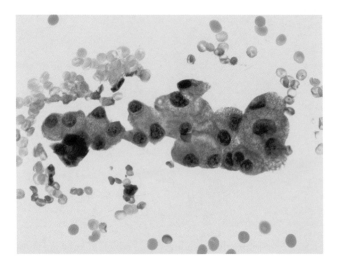

FIGURE 3-34. Another example of foamy gland variant of pancreatic ductal adenocarcinoma. Papanicolaou stain; original magnification, ×400.

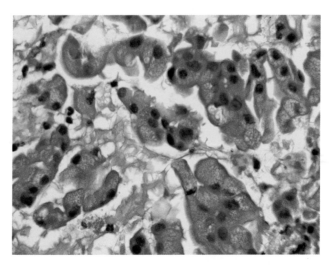

FIGURE 3-35. A cell block preparation with foamy gland adenocarcinoma. Hemotoxylin and eosin stain; original magnification, ×200.

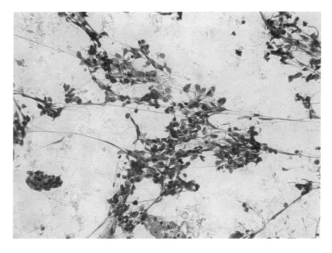

FIGURE 3-36. Small cell carcinoma of the pancreas showing features akin to those of small cell carcinoma of the lung. Papanicolaou stain; original magnification, ×200.

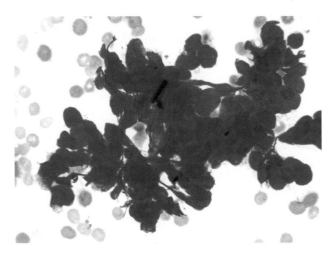

FIGURE 3-37. Small cell carcinoma of the pancreas with abundant nuclear molding. Diff-Quik stain; original magnification, ×400.

variable immunoreactivity with antibodies to neuroendocrine antigens, but most are immunoreactive with antibodies to synaptophysin. Careful clinical and radiographic investigation must be conducted to exclude a metastatic small cell carcinoma from the lung. Although negative TTF-1 immunostaining would favor an extrapulmonary origin, positive staining would not exclude a pancreatic primary as a substantial number of extrapulmonary small cell carcinomas also express TTF-1. Chemotherapy is usually the treatment of choice for small cell carcinoma.

## Ancillary Studies

Most PDAs are immunoreactive with antibodies against CEA and CA19-9. Both markers, however, lack specificity, limiting their use. Half of the PDAs show a cytoplasmic staining with antibodies to CA125. About 80% to 90% of PDAs demonstrate strong and diffuse staining with antibodies to CK7 and about half of the cases show at least focal reactivity with antibodies to CK20. The use of other ancillary studies including both immunocytochemistry and molecular testing for separating benign lesions from PDA will be discussed in the next chapter.

## Differential Diagnosis and Pitfalls

Table 3-4 summarizes the differential diagnosis for aspirates of PDA. Chronic pancreatitis can mimic PDA clinically and radiologically. Further complicating the issue is that chronic pancreatitis and PDA often coexist. Most authors agree that over diagnosis is rarely an issue; however, under diagnosis is more of a problem and likely explains why some studies report the sensitivity of pancreatic FNA to be as low as 60%. The reasons for under diagnosis are likely many in number, but generally include both sampling and interpretive issues. PDA can induce marked desmoplasia and, as was mentioned, can coexist with extensive chronic pancreatitis. In either case, aspirates can be hypocellular and neoplastic cells can be scarce. Given that some cases of chronic pancreatitis may have some degree of associated pancreatic intraepithelial neoplasia, most pathologists are wary of diagnosing rare atypical cells as unequivocally malignant. This is in spite of the fact that the cytology literature has shown that most pancreatic aspirates that are diagnosed as "suspicious" by cytology are from glands harboring cancers after additional diagnostic studies are performed.

Aside from quantitative issues, qualitative factors can also hinder the prospective diagnosis of PDA by cytology. By aspirate, some well-differentiated PDAs can have very subtle atypia and be difficult to separate from reactive changes. The cytologic features that favor a diagnosis of well-differentiated

TABLE 3-4. Differential diagnosis of pancreatic ductal adenocarcinoma.

Chronic pancreatitis
Other epithelial pancreatic neoplasms
   Acinar cell carcinoma
   Pancreatic endocrine tumor
Metastases

PDA over benign disease, such as chronic pancreatitis, include high cellularity, the presence of one cell type (ductal cells), "drunken honeycomb" arrangement, a greater number of atypical cell groups, and single atypical cells (Table 3-5). With

TABLE 3-5. Distinguishing chronic pancreatitis and well-differentiated pancreatic ductal adenocarcinoma.

| Cytologic features | Chronic pancreatitis | Well-differentiated adenocarcinoma |
|---|---|---|
| Low power | | |
| Cellularity | Variable | Usually cellular |
| Arrangement | Two-dimensional sheets with few single cells if any | Two-dimensional sheets with scattered single cells |
| Background | Clean or inflammatory | Clean, inflammatory, or rarely necrotic |
| Intermediate power | | |
| Cell type | Ductal cells, may be admixed with acinar cells (small clusters or large, fibrotic fragments), islet cells, and fragments of fibrotic stroma | Predominantly ductal cells |
| Organization | Regular honeycomb with a maintenance of polarity | "Drunken honeycomb" with a loss of polarity and a variable amount of nuclear overlap and crowding |
| High power | | |
| Nuclear enlargement | Minimal, usually <2× the size of a red blood cell | Usually >2× the size of a red blood cell |
| Nuclear contours | Smooth and regular | Irregular |
| Chromatin | Evenly distributed and finely granular | Coarse with irregular clumping |
| Nucleoli | Small if present | Usually distinct and sometimes macronucleoli can be seen |
| Mitotic figures | Rare | More frequent, can be atypical |
| Isolated atypical cells | Absent | Variable |

brush samples, the atypia seen with reactive changes can be more severe and thus more difficult to distinguish from well-differentiated PDA. Indeed, this explains how a greater percentage of atypical diagnoses with these specimens are found to be benign at follow-up.

Distinguishing well-differentiated PDA from other epithelial neoplasms of the pancreas, such as acinar cell carcinomas and pancreatic endocrine tumors, can usually be done based solely on morphology; however, immunocytochemistry can be used if necessary (see Chapter 2). Pancreatic ductal adenocarsinomas tend to shed cohesive cell groups and sheets of neoplastic cells. The cells themselves show more atypia and prominent nucleoli than do the other epithelial pancreatic neoplastic lesions. The identification of numerous, single, epithelioid cells, acinar or rosette formation, and the lack of significant nuclear atypia should raise one's suspicion of a diagnosis other than PDA.

Metastases to the pancreas can be indistinguishable from primary PDAs by cytology alone. A history of prior malignancy should alert one to this possibility. The judicious use of ancillary studies, such as immunocytochemistry, may be helpful in certain situations.

## Clinical Management and Prognosis

Complete surgical resection with or without postoperative chemoradiation remains the most effective treatment for localized operable disease and offers the only hope of cure. Recently, the use of neoadjuvant chemotherapy has been investigated. Because it postpones surgery, it may benefit patients by leading to the exclusion of those patients with rapidly progressive disease from surgical resection. It also may provide an opportunity for some patients for resection by downstaging their malignancies. For patients with unresectable and metastatic disease, symptomatic relief can be achieved by palliative bypass surgery, celiac nerve blocks, or other local neurosurgical procedures, radiation therapy, and chemotherapy.

The prognosis for PDA is dismal. For untreated patients, the mean survival time is 3 to 6 months. The mean survival time even after complete surgical resection is not much better and is only 10 to 20 months. The 1-year and 5-year survival rates are 10% and 3%, respectively. Patients with small tumors (<3 cm) that are confined to the pancreas with no or limited (1 or 2 peripancreatic lymph nodes) nodal involvement, and no residual disease after resection have the best outcomes, with 5-year survival rates ranging from 25% to 45%. Some of these patients still die from their disease when follow-up times are lengthened.

## Suggested Reading

Centeno BA. Fine needle aspiration biopsy of the pancreas. Clin Lab Med 1998;18:401–427.

Chang KJ, Nguyen P, Erickson RA, Durbin TE, Katz KD. The clinical utility of endoscopic ultrasound-guided fine-needle aspiration in the diagnosis and staging of pancreatic carcinoma. Gastrointest Endosc 1997;45:387–393.

Cohen MB, Egerter DP, Holly EA, Ahn DK, Miller TR. Pancreatic adenocarcinoma: regression analysis to identify improved cytologic criteria. Diagn Cytopathol 1991;7:341–345.

Eloubeidi MA, Chen VK, Eltoum IA, et al. Endoscopic ultrasound-guided fine needle aspiration biopsy of patients with suspected pancreatic cancer: diagnostic accuracy and acute and 30-day complications. Am J Gastroenterol 2003;98:2663–2668.

Eloubeidi MA, Jhala D, Chhieng DC, et al. Yield of endoscopic ultrasound-guided fine-needle aspiration biopsy in patients with suspected pancreatic carcinoma. Cancer 2003;99:285–292.

Erickson RA, Garza AA. Impact of endoscopic ultrasound on the management and outcome of pancreatic carcinoma. Am J Gastroenterol 2000;95:2248–2254.

Goldstein D, Carroll S, Apte M, Keogh G. Modern management of pancreatic carcinoma. Intern Med J 2004;34:475–481.

Gupta RK, Wakefield SJ. Needle aspiration cytology, immuno-cytochemistry, and electron microscopic study of unusual pancreatic carcinoma with pleomorphic giant cells. Diagn Cytopathol 1992;8:522–527.

Hughes JH, Cohen MB. Fine-needle aspiration of the pancreas. Pathology 1996;4:389–407.

Lin F, Staerkel G. Cytologic criteria for well differentiated adenocarcinoma of the pancreas in fine-needle aspiration biopsy specimens. Cancer 2003;99:44–50.

Mitchell ML, Carney CN. Cytologic criteria for the diagnosis of pancreatic carcinoma. Am J Clin Pathol 1985;83:171–176.

Rahemtullah A, Misdraji J, Pitman MB. Adenosquamous carcinoma of the pancreas: cytologic features in 14 cases. Cancer 2003;99: 372–378.

Robins DB, Katz RL, Evans DB, Atkinson EN, Green L. Fine needle aspiration of the pancreas. In quest of accuracy. Acta Cytol 1995;39:1–10.

Silverman JF, Dabbs DJ, Finley JL, Geisinger KR. Fine-needle aspiration biopsy of pleomorphic (giant cell) carcinoma of the pancreas. Cytologic, immunocytochemical, and ultrastructural findings. Am J Clin Pathol 1988;89:714–720.

Stelow EB, Pambuccian SE, Bardales RH, et al. The cytology of pancreatic foamy gland adenocarcinoma. Am J Clin Pathol 2004;121:893–897.

# 4
# Ancillary Testing for the Diagnosis of Pancreatic Ductal Adenocarcinoma

Over the last decade, the molecular biology of pancreatic ductal adenocarcinoma (PDA) has been the subject of intense investigation. As a result, our understanding of the pathogenesis of PDA has significantly advanced. This chapter discusses some of these advances and how they and other developments have facilitated ancillary testing of cytologic samples for the diagnosis of PDA.

## Carcinogenesis of Pancreatic Ductal Carcinoma

The current model of pancreatic carcinogenesis suggests multistep progression, similar to that seen with colorectal carcinogenesis (Figure 4-1). Preinvasive lesions arise within the ductal system and are termed pancreatic intraepithelial neoplasia (PanIN). Recent consensus conferences have categorized these lesions histologically based on current molecular evidence as PanIN 1A, PanIN 1B, PanIN 2, and PanIN 3. Each different lesion represents a step further toward invasive PDA with worsening degrees of cytologic and architectural atypia. The morphologic changes are accompanied by molecular mutations that include the activation of oncogenes and inactivation of tumor suppressor genes.

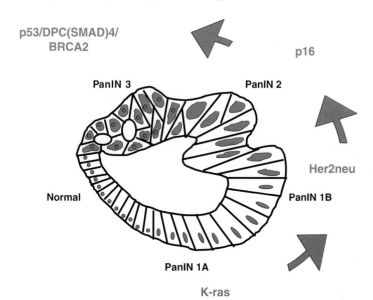

FIGURE 4-1. Model of pancreatic ductal adenocarcinoma (PDA) neogenesis.

## *Oncogenes*

The most common oncogene that is activated in PDA is *k-ras*. K-ras is a signal transduction protein with intrinsic GTPase activity. It binds to GTP and activates a number of downstream effector cascades (e.g., RAF/MARK pathway). After signaling, GTP is hydrolyzed to GDP which turns off K-ras signaling. Mutated *k-ras* synthesizes proteins with altered GTPase activity, resulting in constitutive activation of K-ras. About 90% of PDAs demonstrate *k-ras* point mutations, most of which occur in codon 12 of the *k-ras* gene. The mutation is believed to occur early, and most low-grade intraepithelial lesions (PanIN 1A and 1B) have been found to have the mutation. While the mutation appears to be important for the development of PDA, it is certainly not sufficient. Indeed, PanIN, especially PanIN 1A and 1B, is found commonly in pancreata resected for other tumors or chronic pancreatitis and has been identified frequently in autopsy specimens with otherwise unremarkable pancreata.

The *HER2/neu* oncogene encodes a transmembrane protein with tyrosine kinase activity. This oncogene has been shown to be overexpressed at the protein and mRNA level in some cases of PDA and PanIN. Unlike breast cancer, DNA amplification has been identified only very infrequently. The etiologies of the increased Her2/neu protein and mRNA expressions are thus unclear. As with *k-ras* mutations, Her2/neu overexpression appears to develop early in cancer neogenesis.

## Tumor Suppressor Genes

The inactivation of tumor suppressor genes plays a key role in the initiation and/or progression of many human cancers, including PDA. Currently, *p53*, *DPC4*, and *p16* are known to be the most frequently mutated tumor suppressor genes in PDA. Other tumor suppressor genes that have been infrequently shown to be lost in cases of PDA include *BRCA2*, *MKK4*, *LKB1/STK11*, *ALK5*, and *TGF BR2*.

p16, a member of the family of cyclin-dependent kinase inhibitors, is a tumor suppressor that inhibits the phosphorylation of the retinoblastoma protein, which in turn prohibits cell cycle progression beyond the G1/S restriction point. Inactivation of *p16* gene either by mutation, deletion, or hypermethylation, results in reduced expression of p16 protein and increased cellular proliferation. Loss of p16 function is observed in the majority (95%) of PDAs and has been observed often in PanIN 2. A familiar syndrome associated with the development of melanomas secondary to germline *p16* mutations (familial atypical multiple mole melanoma or FAMMM) is associated with increased risk for the development of PDA.

p53 is a tumor suppressor protein that performs a number of functions, including the induction of apoptosis and cellular growth arrest. Loss of protein function thus leads to increased cell cycling and immortalization. *p53* mutations have been noted in 50% to 75% of PDAs and some cases of PanIN 3. Ironically, molecular mutations of the *p53* gene lead to protein accumulation as the aberrant protein, while nonfunctional, is broken down by the cell less efficiently.

Loss of the tumor suppressor DPC4 (*D*eleted in *P*ancreatic *C*arcinoma locus *4*) or SMAD4 has been noted in slightly more than half (55%) of the PDAs and some cases of PanIN 3. Transforming growth factor-beta (TGF-β) signals through DPC4 protein and arrests the cell in G1. Thus, mutations of the *DPC4* gene lead to an inability for the cell to arrest its cycle.

*BRCA2* mutations are infrequent but are found in a small number of PDAs and PanIN 3 lesions. Furthermore, patients with germline mutations of *BRCA2* are at increased risk for the development of PDA. The BRCA2 protein works in conjunction with the RAD51 protein to repair DNA.

## Other Molecular Abnormalities

Microsatellite instability (MSI) resulting from inactivation of one or more DNA mismatch repair genes is seen in a small proportion of PDAs. When present, MSI is associated with a distinct "medullary" histology characterized by a lack of gland formation with, instead, a syncytial growth pattern, pushing tumor borders, a lymphocytic infiltrate, and extensive tumor necrosis. It has been suggested that PDAs with "medullary" histology and MSI have better prognoses than conventional PDAs. Patients with hereditary nonpolyposis colon cancer are at increased risk for the development of PDA.

## Proteins

The differential expression of a number of proteins has been compared in normal/reactive ductal cells, PanIN, and invasive PDAs. A number of proteins, especially mucins, have been investigated using immunohistochemistry. Recently, additional protein markers overexpressed in PDA have been identified using mRNA microarray technology.

A number of studies have shown that coincident with the neoplastic transformation of the pancreatic ductal epithelium is a change in the expression of particular mucins. Studied mucins include MUC1, MUC2, MUC4, and MUC5a. While normal ductal epithelium does not show much expression of any of these mucins, some of the mucins, particularly MUC1 and MUC4, are overexpressed in conventional PDAs. MUC2 expression is not seen with most PDAs but has been noted in mucinous (colloid) PDAs and some intraductal papillary mucinous neoplasms.

Recent studies with high-throughput or global gene expression profiling have led to the discovery of a number of new biomarkers of PDA. Meosthelin and prostate stem cell antigen (PSCA) are two such examples. Mesothelin is a 40 kDa membrane-bound glycoprotein that may play a role in cell—cell interaction. By mRNA analysis and immunohistochemistry, mesothelin is not expressed in normal pancreatic tissue but is overexpressed in over 90% of PDAs and in high-grade PanIN lesions. Prostate stem cell antigen is also a membrane-bound glycoprotein that is overexpressed in 60% of PDAs but not in non-neoplastic epithelium. It appears to be expressed earlier in PDA neogenesis and has been noted in lower grades of PanIN than mesothelin.

# Ancillary Testing of Cytologic Samples for Molecular Abnormalities

Ancillary testing of cytologic samples for molecular abnormalities can be performed by a number of methods. Ideally, the test should be inexpensive, simple, and use readily available material and laboratory functions. For this reason, immunocytochemistry is often the preferred method. Not all molecular changes allow for such testing, however.

## *Oncogenes*

Testing for *k-ras* mutations requires DNA amplification using polymerase chain reaction (PCR) and then sequencing. Fortunately, most *k-ras* mutations occur at a specific site and only a small area around codon 12 is usually amplified. Studies have reported using *k-ras* mutational analysis with both bile duct brushings and fine needle aspiration (FNA) specimens. The reported sensitivities and specificities vary widely and have ranged from 43% to 77% and from 83% to 100% for bile duct brushings and FNA, respectively. When compared directly with cytology, most studies have shown relatively similar function, suggesting that most false-negative results are secondary to sampling issues. A few studies have shown the molecular testing to be superior to cytology, raising question about the incidence of false-negative cytology secondary to interpretative errors.

Her2/neu overexpression can be shown using immunohistochemistry to gauge protein expression or with methods for mRNA quantification. As the protein and mRNA overexpression has not been shown to be secondary to an increased copy number of the gene, DNA-based methods, such as fluorescent in situ hybridization, would not be applicable. Her2/neu assessment has not been used as an ancillary method with cytology specimens from the pancreas.

## Tumor Suppressor Genes

Although a number of tumor suppressor genes have been shown to be inactivated in cases of PDA, only a few are so consistently inactivated as to be potentially useful for ancillary testing of pancreatic cytologic samples (Table 4-1). These include *p53*, *p16*, and *DPC4/smad4*. Although molecular

TABLE 4-1. Function of immunocytochemistry for the diagnosis of pancreatic ductal adenocarcinoma (PDA).

| Biomarkers | Sensitivity | Specificity | Number of cases reported |
|---|---|---|---|
| p53 | 48% | 97% | 94 |
| DPC4 | 21% | 100% | 94 |
| p16 | 82% | 73% | 39 |
| MUC1 | 96% | 94% | 39 |
| Mesothelin | 68%–100% | 91%–95% | 73 |
| PSCA | 84% | 91% | 30 |

testing for such abnormalities is possible with loss of hetero-zygosity studies, etc., immunocytochemistry is generally used with antibodies to each gene's respective protein. While samples from PDA will generally show loss of expression of p16 and DPC4/smad4, p53 expression will be increased as the mutated protein is less efficiently broken down by the cell. A number of studies have examined the use of immunocyto-chemistry for these proteins as an ancillary method for the diagnosis of PDA. Used individually or in concert, such ancil-lary testing usually shows results comparable or inferior to cytology alone.

## Other Proteins

As was mentioned, a number of other proteins have been shown to be expressed differently in PDA than in non-neoplastic ductal epithelium. These include MUC1, MUC2, MUC4, prostate stem cell antigen, and mesothelin, among others. A number of studies have been published using immu-nocytochemistry with pancreatic cytologic samples and have, in general, shown results similar to cytology alone (Table 4-1). The authors of these studies usually note that such testing may prove helpful in selected cases.

## Other Tests, Future Directions

A number of other molecular tests may come to be more easily and widely used and could prove to be of assistance for diag-nosing PDA with cytology samples. One example is the TRAP (telomeric repeat amplification protocol) assay that evaluates telomerase activity. Telomerase activity is generally increased in most cancers and has been shown to be increased in PDA. The RNA-coupled enzyme stabilizes the telomere length of chromosomes and is thus implicated in cellular immortality.

It has recently been shown that FNA can provide sufficient material for global gene expression profiling. Such testing may prove helpful for diagnosis or may provide further prog-nostic and treatment information. Testing of the pancreas using cytology samples would be ideal as most tumors are not resectable when they come to clinical attention.

## Suggested Reading

Chhieng DC, Benson E, Eltoum I, et al. MUC1 and MUC2 expression in pancreatic ductal carcinoma obtained by fine-needle aspiration. Cancer 2003;99:365–371.

Giorgadze TA, Peterman H, Baloch ZW, et al. Diagnostic utility of mucin profile in fine-needle aspiration specimens of the pancreas: an immunohistochemical study with surgical pathology correlation. Cancer 2006;108:186–197.

Jhala N, Jhala D, Vickers SM, et al. Biomarkers in diagnosis of pancreatic carcinoma in fine-needle aspirates. Am J Clin Pathol 2006;126:572–579.

Lapkus O, Gologan O, Liu Y, et al. Determination of sequential mutation accumulation in pancreas and bile duct brushing cytology. Mod Pathol 2006;19:907–913.

Maitra A, Adsay NV, Argani P, et al. Multicomponent analysis of the pancreatic adenocarcinoma progression model using a pancreatic intraepithelial neoplasia tissue microarray. Mod Pathol 2003;16:902–912.

McCarthy DM, Maitra A, Argani P, et al. Novel markers of pancreatic adenocarcinoma in fine-needle aspiration: mesothelin and prostate stem cell antigen labeling increases accuracy in cytologically borderline cases. Appl Immunohistochem Mol Morphol 2003;11:238–243.

Saxby AJ, Nielsen A, Scarlett CJ, et al. Assessment of HER-2 status in pancreatic adenocarcinoma: correlation of immunohistochemistry, quantitative real-time RT-PCR, and FISH with aneuploidy and survival. Am J Surg Pathol 2005;29:1125–1133.

Tada M, Komatsu Y, Kawabe T, et al. Quantitative analysis of K-ras gene mutation in pancreatic tissue obtained by endoscopic ultrasonography-guided fine needle aspiration: clinical utility for diagnosis of pancreatic tumor. Am J Gastroenterol 2002;97:2263–2270.

Wilentz RE, Goggins M, Redston M, et al. Genetic, immunohistochemical, and clinical features of medullary carcinoma of the pancreas: a newly described and characterized entity. Am J Pathol 2000;156:1641–1651.

van Heek T, Rader AE, Offerhaus GJ, et al. K-ras, p53, and DPC4 (MAD4) alterations in fine-needle aspirates of the pancreas: a molecular panel correlates with and supplements cytologic diagnosis. Am J Clin Pathol 2002;117:755–765.

# 5
# Acinar Cell Carcinoma

Acinar cell carcinoma (ACC) is a rare malignant epithelial neoplasm of the exocrine pancreas. It mostly affects older individuals; however, it can occur in individuals of any age, from 3 to 90 years. It is slightly more common in men. The neoplasms most often arise in the head of the pancreas and may have developed both lymph node and liver metastases at time of diagnosis. Most patients present with nonspecific abdominal complaints, and biliary obstruction is uncommon. Rarely, patients may display symptoms associated with increased serum levels of pancreatic enzymes, such as distal fat necrosis or arthralgias.

Grossly, ACCs tend to be more circumscribed than pancreatic ductal adenocarcinomas (PDAs) and have pushing rather than infiltrative borders. These features are seen histologically, as well. ACCs also do not induce prominent desmoplasia. The neoplastic cells are arranged in acini, sheets, trabeculae, or glandular structures. The individual cells may show varying degrees of differentiation, but typically have abundant, granular cytoplasm. Nuclear pleomorphism tends to be less than that seen with PDAs; however, prominent nucleoli are usually seen. Immunohistochemistry can be used to confirm acinar cell differentiation; tumors typically react with antibodies to trypsin, chymotrypsin, and lipase. It should be noted that these tumors can show both ductal and endocrine differentiation that may be noted both histologically and by immunohistochemistry.

## General Diagnostic Approach

These tumors usually appear as solid masses by imaging and only rarely appear cystic. Aspirates are usually cellular and the initial differential diagnosis generally includes other epithelioid pancreatic neoplasms such as pancreatic endocrine tumor (PET), solid-pseudopapillary neoplasm (SPPN), and PDA. When these tumors arise in young patients, pancreatoblastoma should be considered in the differential diagnosis. Cytologic clues may be helpful for narrowing the differential diagnosis; however, without immunocytochemistry, a definitive diagnosis is often difficult to make.

## Diagnostic Criteria

The cytologic features of ACC recapitulate those seen by histology (Table 5-1). Aspirates are usually very cellular and consist of both single cells and loose clusters (Figure 5-1). Rarely, more sheetlike structures may be seen (Figure 5-2). The background is not as "dirty" as that seen with PDA and, instead, numerous naked nuclei are usually seen (Figures 5-3 and 5-4). Small clusters of cells often show conspicuous acinar formation (Figures 5-5, 5-6, and 5-7), although this can be confused with the pseudorosette formation seen in aspirates of PETs. The individual cells have indistinct cells borders and abundant granular cytoplasm (Figure 5-8). Nuclei may be centrally or eccentrically placed and binucleation can rarely be seen (Figure 5-9). The nuclei have irregular nuclear

TABLE 5-1. Cytologic features of acinar cell carcinoma.

Overall characteristics
  Cellular aspirate with single cells and loose clusters with the formation of acini
Background
  No necrosis or debris
  Naked nuclei
Neoplastic cells
  Abundant granular cytoplasm with indistinct cell borders
  Atypical central or eccentric nuclei with prominent nucleoli

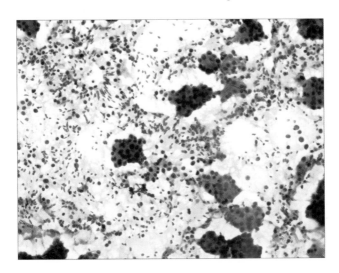

FIGURE 5-1. Aspirates from acinar cell carcinoma are usually very cellular and consist of both loose clusters and numerous single cells. Papanicolaou stain; original magnification, ×40.

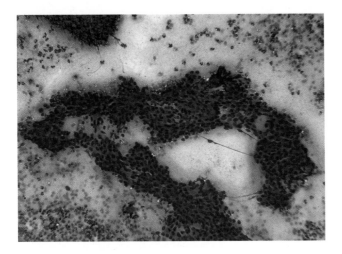

FIGURE 5-2. Large tissue fragments can also be seen with acinar cell carcinoma. Diff-Quik stain; original magnification, ×40.

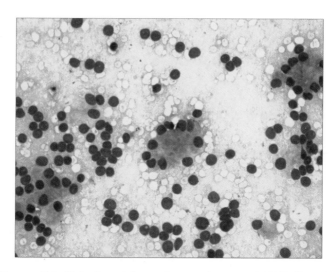

FIGURE 5-3. Naked nuclei are frequently seen. Diff-Quik stain; original magnification, ×100.

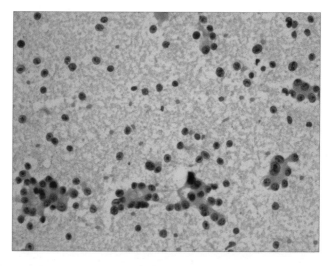

FIGURE 5-4. Another example of acinar cell carcinoma with abundant naked nuclei in a granular background. Papanicolaou stain; original magnification, ×100.

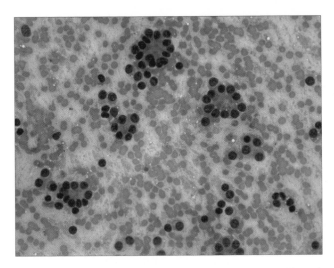

FIGURE 5-5. Acinar formation is usually seen in acinar cell carcinomas and can be confused with the rosette formation seen in pancreatic endocrine tumors. Diff-Quik stain; original magnification, ×100.

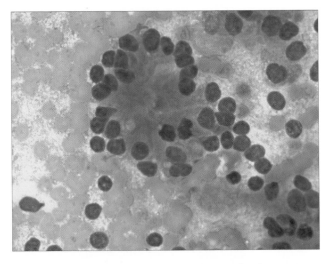

FIGURE 5-6. Acinar formation mimics a neuroendocrine tumor, warranting immunohistochemistry for identification. Diff-Quik stain; original magnification, ×200.

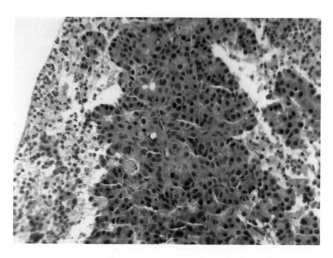

FIGURE 5-7. Acinar formation can also easily be appreciated in cell block preparations. Hemotoxylin and eosin stain; original magnification, ×40.

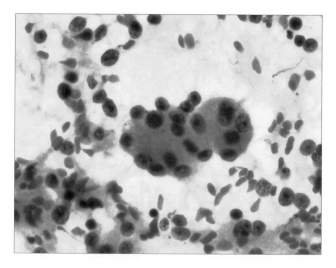

FIGURE 5-8. The individual cells have indistinct borders and abundant granular cytoplasm. Nuclei may be centrally or eccentrically placed. Papanicolaou stain; original magnification, ×400.

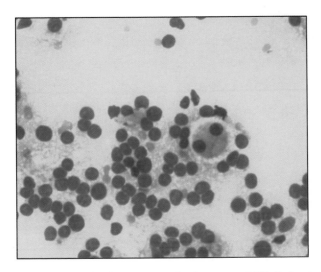

FIGURE 5-9. Binucleation can rarely be seen. Diff-Quik stain; original magnification, ×100.

contours, clumped chromatin (Figure 5-10), and, usually, a single prominent nucleolus (Figure 5-11). Anisonucleosis is often present but usually of a much lesser degree than that seen with PDAs (Figure 5-12).

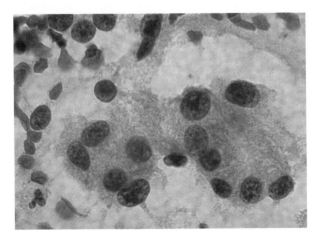

FIGURE 5-10. The nuclei often have clumped chromatin. Papanicolaou stain; original magnification, ×600.

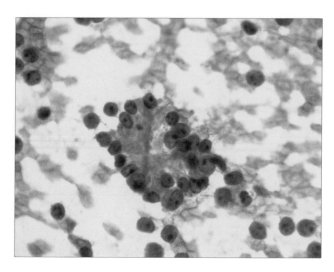

FIGURE 5-11. Single prominent nucleoli are noted in this group of neoplastic acinar cells. Papanicolaou stain; original magnification, ×400.

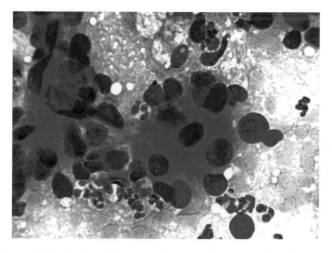

FIGURE 5-12. Anisonucleosis can be seen but is usually of a lesser degree than that of pancreatic ductal adenocarcinoma. Diff-Quik stain; original magnification, ×400.

# Differential Diagnosis and Pitfalls
(Table 5-2)

The most common differential diagnosis to be considered with aspirates of ACCs will be PET. Aspirates from both are cellular with numerous single cells and loose clusters. Both may show prominent acinar or pseudorosette formation and have abundant background naked nuclei. Although ACCs tend to have more nuclear atypia and prominent nucleoli, both features, as well as abundant granular cytoplasm, can be seen in PETs. Because of the overlap in the cytologic features of these two lesions, immunocytochemistry is recommended for their distinction.

Aspirates from pancreatoblastomas may show overlapping cytologic and immunocytochemical features with ACCs. The presence of squamous or stromal elements may be used to help distinguish the two. Fortunately, the neoplasms tend to be restricted to different patient ages. Indeed, tumors that histologically appear to be ACCs in children are noted to behave more akin to pancreatoblastomas and vice versa.

Most SPPNs and PDAs can be distinguished cytologically from ACCs. Solid-pseudopapillary neoplasms occur almost exclusively in women, tend to be composed of a smaller, more monotonous cell population, and have metachromatic stromal material. Aspirates from PDAs do not show acinar formation and demonstrate more marked cytologic atypia and necrosis.

Rarely, the differential diagnosis may include normal pancreatic parenchyma and heterotopic pancreatic tissue (when occurring outside the pancreas). Aspirates from normal

TABLE 5-2. Differential diagnosis for aspirates from acinar cell carcinoma.

Pancreatic endocrine tumor
Solid-pseudopapillary neoplasm
Ductal adenocarcinoma, especially undifferentiated variety
Pancreatoblastoma
Normal pancreatic parenchyma

pancreatic parenchyma display more cohesive cell groups, well-defined acini, and a lack of cytologic atypia (Figures 5-13 and 5-14). In addition, ductal cells are usually also present.

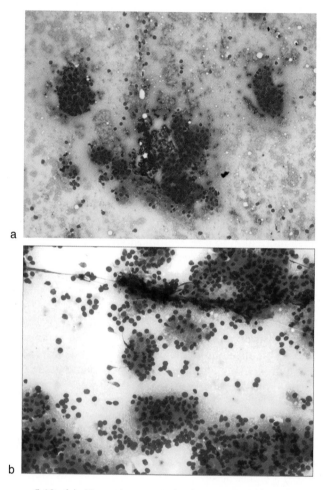

FIGURE 5-13. (a) Normal pancreatic tissue showing well-formed acini. Diff-Quik stain; original magnification, ×40. (b) Acinar cell carcinoma with large tissue fragments, acini and numerous naked nuclei. Diff-Quik stain; original magnification, ×40.

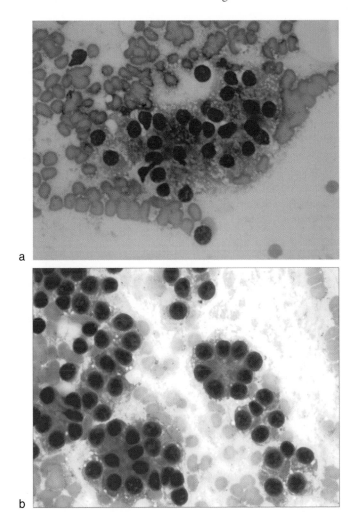

FIGURE 5-14. (a) Benign acinar cells with small, round, uniform nuclei, abundant granular cytoplasm without prominent nucleoli. Diff-Quik stain; original magnification, ×400. (b) Neoplastic acinar cells with nuclear enlargement and increased nuclear–cytoplasmic ratio. Diff-Quik stain; original magnification, ×400.

## Ancillary Testing

Acinar cell carcinomas rarely are confused for non-neoplastic entities and, thus, most ancillary testing has been used to separate these neoplasms from other pancreatic neoplasms. Acinar cell carcinomas express strong immunoreactivity with antibodies to cytokeratin and pancreatic enzyme antigens. They do not typically show immunoreactivity with antibodies to endocrine antigens such as synaptophysin or chromogranin, and if any immunoreactivity is present, it tends to be limited to occasional cells with weak staining. Please refer to Table 2-3 for the differential diagnosis based on immunocytochemistry.

It should also be noted that specific molecular or other tests used to distinguish aspirates of PDAs from those from non-neoplastic lesions will usually not be of assistance with aspirates from ACCs. Acinar cell carcinomas do not develop via the same molecular pathway as PDAs and do not have the same molecular abnormalities, such as *k-ras* mutations. Thus, *k-ras* mutational analysis will not be useful for identifying these tumors.

## Clinical Management and Prognosis

Acinar cell carcinomas behave poorly and only marginally better than PDAs with a 5-year survival of approximately 6%. Surgical resection offers the only hope for cure and is often considered for low stage disease. The chemotherapeutic regimen used is similar to that for PDA and thus distinguishing these lesions from PETs is important, as it may instigate a potentially different chemotherapy regime than that used for PETs. As PETs show so many overlapping cytologic features, yet have different prognoses and treatment regimens, we recommend immunocytochemistry be performed to arrive at a definitive diagnosis, particularly when the patient is not a surgical candidate.

# Suggested Reading

Klimstra DS, Heffess CS, Oertel JE, Rosai J. Acinar cell carcinoma of the pancreas. A clinicopathologic study of 28 cases. Am J Surg Pathol 1992;16:815–837.

Klimstra DS, Longnecker D. Acinar cell carcinoma. In: Hamilton SR, Aaltonen LA, eds. Pathology and genetics of tumours of the digestive system. France, Lyon: IARC Press; 2000:241–243.

Labate AM, Klimstra DL, Zakowski MF. Comparative cytologic features of pancreatic acinar cell carcinoma and islet cell tumor. Diagn Cytopathol 1997;16:112–116.

Stelow EB, Bardales RH, Shami VM, et al. Cytology of pancreatic acinar cell carcinoma. Diagn Cytopathol 2006;34:367–372.

# 6
# Pancreatoblastoma

Pancreatoblastoma is extremely rare and represents 0.5% of all pancreatic epithelial tumors. It primarily occurs in children 10 years of age or younger, although cases in adults have been reported. There is a slight male predominance. Patients usually present with an abdominal mass with or without nonspecific symptoms such as pain and weight loss. Jaundice is notably uncommon. About one third of patients have elevated serum levels of alpha-fetoprotein (AFP). Radiologic examination often reveals a well-demarcated, heterogeneous mass. Calcification is not unusual.

## Diagnostic Approach

Pancreatoblastomas present as solid masses and should top the list of potential diagnoses for a pancreatic mass in a child in his or her first year of life. It should be easy to distinguish pancreatoblastoma from normal pancreas and pancreatic ductal adenocarcinoma (PDA). Cytologically, the main challenge is to distinguish this entity from other epithelioid neoplasms of the pancreas or other childhood neoplasms. When pancreatoblastoma is suspected, attempts should be made to obtain additional material for ancillary studies.

TABLE 6-1. Cytologic features of pancreatoblastoma.

Cellular
Biphasic with epithelial and stromal components
Epithelial component
    Three-dimensional syncytial groups of intermediate-to-large
        pleomorphic cells
    Acinar structures composed of cells with more abundant cytoplasm and
        prominent nucleoli
    Squamoid corpuscles
Stromal component
    Primitive spindle-shaped cells
    Heterologous stroma, e.g., cartilage

## Cytologic Findings

Aspirates of pancreatoblastomas are usually highly cellular. Most reports of these cases stress the presence of biphasic cellular components (Table 6-1; Figure 6-1). The mesenchymal component is composed of primitive spindle-shaped cells (Figure 6-2). Heterologous elements, such as cartilage, can

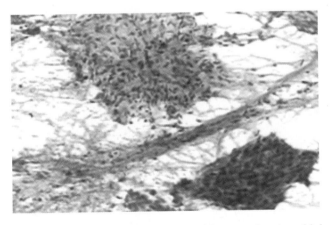

FIGURE 6-1. Cellular smear of a pancreatoblastoma showing a biphasic pattern with both epithelial (lower right corner) and stromal elements (upper left corner). Ultrafast Papanicolaou stain; original magnification, ×40.

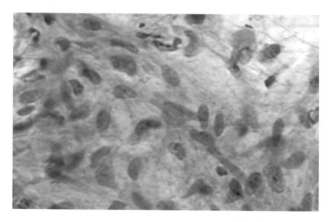

FIGURE 6-2. Stromal component composed of atypical, primitive spindle cells. Ultrafast Papanicolaou stain; original magnification, ×400.

sometimes be seen. The epithelial component consists of three-dimensional syncytial groups of intermediate-to-large pleomorphic cells (Figure 6-3). Acinar structures can be seen and are composed of cells with more abundant granular cytoplasm and prominent nucleoli. Squamoid corpuscles have

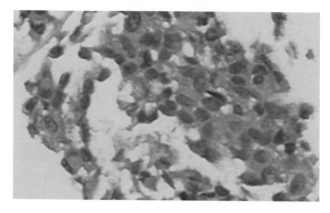

FIGURE 6-3. Cell block preparation showing the epithelial component of a pancreatoblastoma, a syncytial group of large pleomorphic cells. Hemotoxylin and eosin stain; original magnification, ×400.

been described and are composed of large epithelial cells with abundant pale cytoplasm that form swirling eddies. Both acinar structures and squamoid corpuscles are more readily appreciated with cell block preparations.

## Differential Diagnosis and Pitfalls

Table 6-2 summarizes the differential diagnosis of pancreatoblastoma. Because the presence of both epithelial and heterologous stromal components in a pancreatic mass is unusual for other primary pancreatic neoplasms, the diagnosis is usually obvious. For those tumors that are stroma poor, the differential diagnosis includes acinar cell carcinoma (ACC), pancreatic endocrine tumor (PET), solid-pseudopapillary neoplasm (SPPN), and PDA. Distinguishing pancreatoblastoma from ACC can be a challenge cytologically as neoplastic cells with acinar differentiation can be seen in both entities. The presence of squamous corpuscles and stromal elements would exclude a diagnosis of ACC. The lack of papillary structures, hyaline globules, and nuclear grooves would preclude a diagnosis of SPPN. The presence of abundant granular cytoplasm, conspicuous cellular pleomorphism, and prominent nucleoli argue against a diagnosis of PET. Pancreatic ductal adenocarcinoma is rarely considered as it is improbable in pediatric patients and usually demonstrates

TABLE 6-2. Differential diagnosis of pancreatoblastoma.

Other primary pancreatic neoplasms
    Pancreatic ductal adenocarcinoma
    Solid pseudopapillary neoplasm
    Pancreatic endocrine tumor
    Acinar cell carcinoma
Other childhood malignances
    Wilms tumor
    Neuroblastoma
    Malignant lymphoma
    Other

sheets and clusters of epithelial cells with significant pleomorphism. Immunocytochemistry will allow for the distinction of
those neoplasms other than ACC and pancreatoblastoma.

In addition to primary pancreatic neoplasms, one should
also consider other childhood malignancies, such as Wilms
tumor, neuroblastoma, and malignant lymphoma, in children
with large upper abdominal or retroperitoneal masses. The
findings of squamous corpuscles, acinar structures, and heterologous elements argue for a diagnosis of pancreatoblastoma. When the tumor is inoperable and chemotherapy is
contemplated, it is prudent to perform immunocytochemistry
or other ancillary studies to arrive at a definitive diagnosis
because the therapeutic regimes may be different for non-
pancreatic tumors, such as Wilms tumor, that can also show
mixed elements.

## Ancillary Studies (Table 6-3)

Except for the squamous corpuscles, the epithelial component typically demonstrates strong immunoreactivity with
antibodies to CAM 5.2 and pancreatic exocrine enzymes such
as lipase, trypsin, chymotrypsin, and alpha-1-antitrypsin, but
not with antibodies to alpha-amylase. Immunoreactivity
with antibodies to neuroendocrine markers can be seen in

TABLE 6-3. Immunoprofile of pancreatoblastoma.

| |
| --- |
| Usually diffusely positive |
|    CAM 5.2 |
|    Pancreatic enzymes—lipase, trypsin, chymotrypsin, and alpha-1-antitrypsin, but not alpha-amylase |
| Sometimes positive |
|    Alpha-fetoprotein |
|    CEA |
|    CA19-9 |
| Scattered cells positive |
|    Neuroendocrine markers—chromogranin A and synaptophysin |

Staining with the above markers is mainly observed in the epithelial component but not in the squamoid corpuscles or stromal components.

scattered cells. Some tumors also demonstrate immunoreactivity with antibodies to AFP, CEA, and CA19-9.

## Clinical Management and Prognosis

Surgical resection is the mainstay of treatment for pancreatoblastoma. Chemotherapy and radiotherapy may be beneficial to patients with recurrent, residual, unresectable, or metastatic disease. The overall 5-year survival is 50%. In pediatric patients without metastatic disease at the time of presentation, the 5-year survival is 65%. In pediatric patients with metastasis and adult patients, however, the prognosis is poor and the mean survival time is 18 months and 10 months, respectively. Indeed, adult pancreatoblastomas behave much more like ACC than they do like pancreatoblastomas of childhood, leading some to wonder if pancreatoblastomas should be considered as a distinct diagnostic entity in adult patients.

## Acknowledgment

We would like to thank Dr. Grace Yang, Weill Medical College of Cornell University, New York, NY, for the photomicrographs of a pancreablastoma.

## *Suggested Reading*

Dhebri AR, Connor S, Campbell F, Ghaneh P, Sutton R, Neoptolemos JP. Diagnosis, treatment and outcome of pancreatoblastoma. Pancreatology 2004;4:441–451; discussion 452–453.

Hasegawa Y, Ishida Y, Kato K, et al. Pancreatoblastoma. A case report with special emphasis on squamoid corpuscles with optically clear nuclei rich in biotin. Acta Cytol 2003;47:679–684.

Henke AC, Kelley CM, Jensen CS, Timmerman TG. Fine-needle aspiration cytology of pancreatoblastoma. Diagn Cytopathol 2001;25:118–121.

Klimstra DS, Wenig BM, Adair CF, Heffess CS. Pancreatoblastoma.
A clinicopathologic study and review of the literature. Am J Surg
Pathol 1995;19:1371–1389.

Pitman MB, Faquin WC. The fine-needle aspiration biopsy cytology
of pancreatoblastoma. Diagn Cytopathol 2004;31:402–406.

Zhu LC, Sidhu GS, Cassai ND, Yang GC. Fine-needle aspiration
cytology of pancreatoblastoma in a young woman: report of a case
and review of the literature. Diagn Cytopathol 2005;33:258–262.

# 7
# Solid-Pseudopapillary Neoplasm

Also known as solid-cystic tumor, papillary-cystic tumor, and solid and papillary tumor of the pancreas, this low-grade primary pancreatic epithelial neoplasm accounts for 1% of all exocrine pancreatic neoplasms. It occurs predominantly in adolescent girls and young women and is rare in men and children. Patients often present with vague abdominal discomfort/pain and an enlarging abdominal mass. Not infrequently, patients are asymptomatic and the tumors are found incidentally on physical examination or by imaging for the workup for unrelated conditions. Jaundice and hormonal disturbances are rare. Ultrasound and computed tomography (CT) usually reveal a well-demarcated and variably cystic mass, averaging 10 cm and usually located in the body or tail of the pancreas. Tumor calcification may be present. As smaller tumors are identified with the increased use of more sensitive imaging techniques, cystic degeneration and calcification are often not seen.

## General Diagnostic Approach

Solid-pseudopapillary neoplasms (SPPNs) may appear either primarily solid or cystic radiologically and, as a result, one may start at different points within our algorithms. Unlike true cystic neoplasms of the pancreas, aspirates from the lesions are almost always cellular. Because the neoplastic cells of SPPN appear monotonous and less cohesive when compared to pancreatic ductal adenocarcinomas (PDAs), the cytologist usually has little problem distinguishing the two entities. However, it can be a challenge to distinguish SPPN from other epithelioid neoplasms, such as pancreatic endocrine tumors (PETs). Because significant overlap of cytologic features is often noted among these lesions and specific therapy may depend upon the diagnosis, one should be wary to give a definitive diagnosis without ancillary studies. In equivocal cases, one may choose to render a less definitive diagnosis such as "epithelioid neoplasm" and discuss the differential diagnosis in a note.

## Diagnostic Criteria

Aspirates from these neoplasms are usually cellular and show characteristic cytologic findings (Table 7-1). However, when only cystically degenerated areas are sampled, the smears may rarely be paucicellular and contain predominantly proteinaeous fluid and/or necrotic debris, which may then result in a false-negative diagnosis. Neoplastic cells are arranged singly, in loosely cohesive clusters and in linear and branching papillary structures (Figures 7-1, 7-2, and 7-3). The latter, resembling Chinese calligraphy, have fibrovascular cores lined by one or more layers of neoplastic cells (Figure 7-4).

TABLE 7-1. Cytologic features of solid-pseudopapillary neoplasm.

Highly cellular aspirates
Single cells, loose clusters, and branching papillary fronds
Monotonous and bland cells
Clefted nuclei (or nuclear grooves)
Myxoid and metachromatic stroma and background material
Rare necrotic debris*

* Necrotic debris is seen rarely when areas of cystic degeneration are sampled.

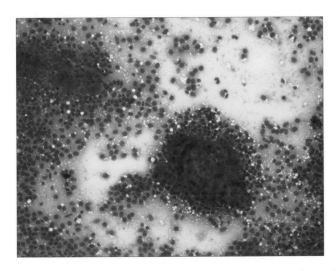

FIGURE 7-1. Aspirates of solid pseudopapillary neoplasm (SPPN) are usually cellular and consist of cells arranged singly and in loosely cohesive clusters. Diff-Quik stain; original magnification, ×20.

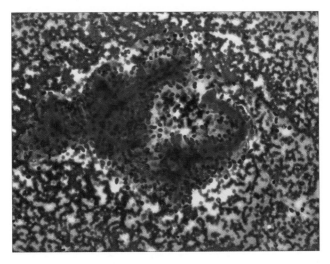

FIGURE 7-2. Large tissue fragments, often papillary with a central capillary, are typical of SPPN. Diff-Quik stain; original magnification, ×40.

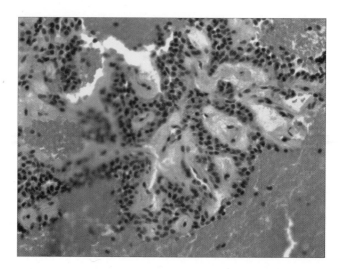

FIGURE 7-3. A branching papillary tissue fragment in a cell block preparation. Hemotoxylin and eosin stain; original magnification, ×40.

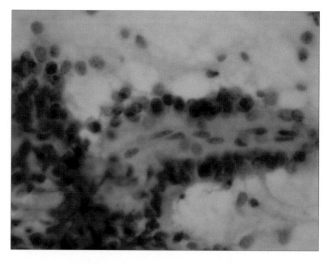

FIGURE 7-4. A papilla with a central fibrovascular core covered by one or more layers of neoplastic cells. Papanicolaou stain; original magnification, ×200.

The stroma of the fibrovascular cores appears myxoid and metachromatic in air-dried, Diff-Quik–stained preparations (Figure 7-5).

Individual cells are uniform and bland (Figures 7-6 and 7-7). The nuclei are round to oval with evenly dispersed or somewhat granular chromatin and small indistinct nucleoli (Figure 7-8). Nuclear grooves are frequently noted. Mitotic figures and nuclear atypia are rarely encountered. The cytoplasm is delicate and can range from scant to moderate (Figure 7-9). The presence of long cytoplasmic processes has been described (Figure 7-10). Another characteristic finding is the presence of metachromatic hyaline globules that are usually located extracellularly but have been noted intracellularly and, rarely, within the lumen of glandular structures (Figures 7-11, 7-12, and 7-13). These globules, as with the stroma within the fibrovascular cores, are periodic acid Schiffs (PAS) positive.

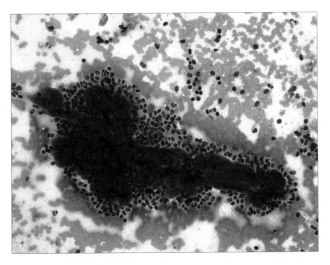

FIGURE 7-5. The stroma of the fibrovascular cores appears myxoid and metachromatic with Diff-Quik stain. Original magnification, ×40.

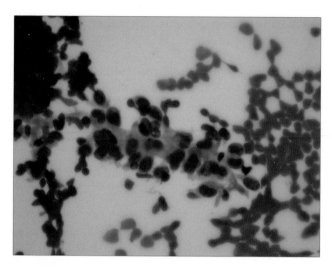

FIGURE 7-6. Individual neoplastic cells are uniform and bland. Papanicolaou stain; original magnification; ×400.

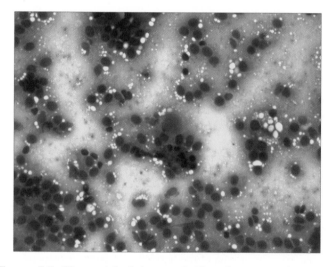

FIGURE 7-7. The nuclei of the neoplastic cells are round to oval. Diff-Quik stain; original magnification; ×100.

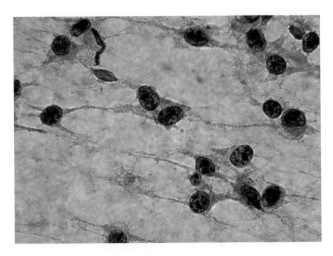

FIGURE 7-8. Individual cells may have somewhat granular chromatin and small indistinct nucleoli. Papanicolaou stain; original magnification, ×400.

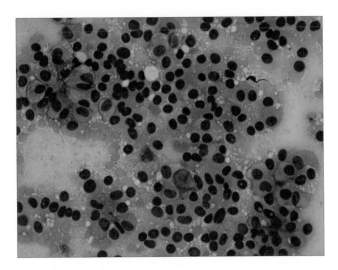

FIGURE 7-9. The cytoplasm is delicate and can range from scant to moderate. Diff-Quik stain; original magnification, ×100.

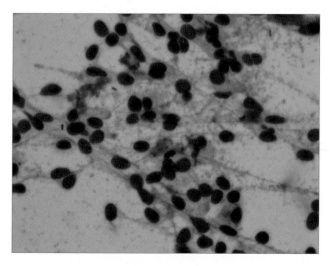

FIGURE 7-10. Long cytoplasmic processes can sometimes be seen. Papanicolaou stain; original magnification, ×200.

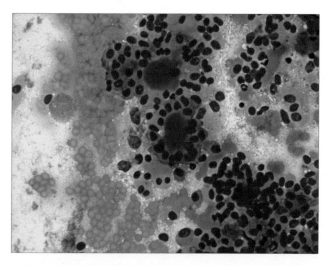

FIGURE 7-11. Extracellular metachromatic hyaline globules are often seen with SPPNs. Diff-Quik stain; original magnification, ×100.

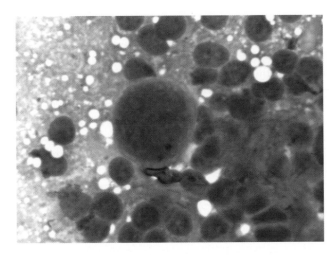

FIGURE 7-12. A hyaline globule with a smooth border and homogeneous appearance. Diff-Quik stain; original magnification, ×400.

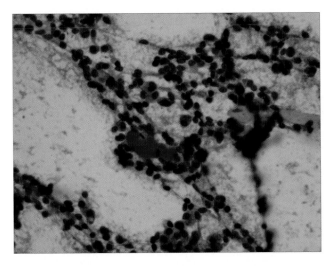

FIGURE 7-13. Hyaline globules can appear orangeophilic in Papanicolaou preparations. Original magnification, ×40.

## Ancillary Studies

The immunoprofile for SPPNs is distinct and can aid in distinguishing these tumors from other pancreatic neoplasms (Table 7-2). Solid-pseudopapillary neoplasms typically do not react with antibodies to cytokeratin, CEA, CA19-9, and some pancreatic enzyme markers, such as trypsin, but do react with antibodies to vimentin, neuron-specific enolase (NSE), CD10, CD56, alpha-1-antitrypsin, and alpha-1-antichymotrypsin (Figure 7-14). The tumors also stain variably with antibodies to synaptophysin, a potential pitfall when differentiating between SPPNs and PETs. Immunoreactivity with antibodies to chromogranin A and other islet cell peptide hormones has not been reported. The tumors are also reactive with antibodies to progesterone receptor, but not estrogen receptor. Recent studies have also shown tumor cells to have nuclear reactivity with antibodies to beta-catenin. Molecular tests used to assist in the diagnosis of PDA will not be helpful with aspirates from these tumors because these tests evaluate molecular changes that are not present in SPPNs.

TABLE 7-2. Immunocytochemistry of solid-pseudopapillary neoplasm.

| Reactive | Nonreactive |
| --- | --- |
| Vimentin | Cytokeratin* |
| Neuron-specific enolase | Chromogranin |
| Progesterone receptor | CEA |
| Beta-catenin | CA19-9 |
| Alpha-1-antitrypsin | Synaptophysin* |
| Alpha-1-antichymotrypsin | Trypsin |
| CD10 | Chymotrypsin |
| CD56 | Amylase |
| | Estrogen receptor |

\* Immunoreactivity with antibodies to various cytokeratins and synaptophysin has been reported, but even when present is not usually diffuse or strong.

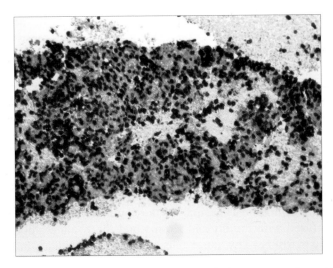

FIGURE 7-14. The tumor cells are strongly immunoreactive with antibodies to vimentin. Cell block; original magnification, ×40.

## Differential Diagnosis and Pitfalls

The differential diagnosis of a pancreatic aspirate showing a relatively uniform cell population should also include PET, acinar cell carcinoma (ACC), and pancreatoblastoma (Table 7-3). Pancreatic endocrine tumors often occur in older patients and can be associated with a variety of clinical syndromes. Rosette or pseudorosette formation, "salt-and-pepper" type chromatin, and the absence of papillary structures and hyaline globules would favor a diagnosis of PET. Acinar cell

TABLE 7-3. Differential diagnosis for solid-pseudopapillary neoplasm.

Monotonous cells
  Pancreatic endocrine tumor
  Acinar cell carcinoma
  Pancreatoblastoma
Cystic lesion with papillae
  Intraductal papillary mucinous neoplasm

carcinoma is more common in older men but can affect patients of varying ages. Aspirates of ACC usually consist of loosely cohesive clusters of neoplastic cells with round-to-oval nuclei, prominent nucleoli, and moderate amount of granular cytoplasm. Acinar structures may be noted, but papillary structures are usually absent. Pancreatoblastoma rarely occurs after the age of 10 years and is more common in boys. The findings of squamous corpuscles and spindled or mesenchymal components are characteristic findings of pancreatoblastoma.

The presence of papillary structures may lead one to consider a diagnosis of intraductal papillary mucinous neoplasm. The mucinous background of these tumors should not be confused with the myxoid stroma and the hyaline globules seen in SPPNs. The tumor cells of intraductal papillary mucinous neoplasms are columnar and may show conspicuous cytologic atypia. The clinical scenario may also provide important clues as intraductal papillary mucinous neoplasms tend to occur in elderly patients, often with histories of chronic pancreatitis.

Solid-pseudopapillary neoplasms should also be distinguished from other cystic lesions, such as pseudocysts, serous cystadenomas, and mucinous cystic neoplasms. Patients with pseudocysts usually have a recent history of pancreatitis and the aspirates consist of inflammatory cells and debris without epithelial cells (except for bowel mucosa inadvertently procured during endoscopic ultrasound-guided fine needle aspiration). Aspirates of serous cystadenomas are paucicellular with a few clusters of bland-appearing cuboidal-to-columnar cells in a proteinaceous background. These often occur in older women.

## Clinical Management and Prognosis

Although the majority (over 95%) of SPPNs behave in a benign fashion, the treatment of choice is surgical resection. Even when the rare case does metastasize, the overall prognosis is good; only rarely do patients die from this tumor.

# *Suggested Reading*

Bardales RH, Centeno B, Mallery JS, et al. Endoscopic ultrasound-guided fine needle aspiration cytology diagnosis of solid-pseudopapillary tumor of the pancreas. Am J Clin Pathol 2004;121:654–662.

Klimstra DS, Wenig BM, Heffess CS. Solid-pseudopapillary tumor of the pancreas: a typically cystic carcinoma of low malignant potential. Semin Diagn Pathol 2000;17:66–80.

Notohara KMD, Hamazaki SMD, Tsukayama CMD, et al. Solid-pseudopapillary tumor of the pancreas: immunohistochemical localization of neuroendocrine markers and CD10. Am J Surg Pathol 2000;24:1361–1371.

Pettinato G, Di Vizia D, Maninvel JC, Pambuccian SE, Somma P, Insabato L. Solid-pseudopapillary tumor of the páncreas—a neoplasm with distinct and highly characteristic nuclear features. Diagn Cytopathol 2002;27:325–334.

# 8
# Pancreatic Endocrine Tumors

Pancreatic endocrine tumors (PETs) are uncommon, accounting for 2% of all pancreatic neoplasms. Previously, it had been noted that somewhere between 60% to 85% of PETs were functioning tumors and were associated with a variety of clinical syndromes (Table 8-1). In today's world, this no longer is true, and PETs often present without clinical syndromes, often identified incidentally by radiologic imaging. Because patients with nonfunctioning PETs are either asymptomatic or present with nonspecific symptoms, fine needle aspiration (FNA) is often employed as a diagnostic test. It can also be used to establish a diagnosis of metastatic disease.

Pancreatic endocrine tumors can occur at any age but are more common in older adults. There is no sex predilection. The tumors may also occur in association with a variety of hereditary syndromes, including multiple endocrine neoplasia type I and von Hippel Lindau syndrome.

Tumors can develop anywhere within the pancreas but most frequently involve the pancreatic tail. Radiologically, PETs are well circumscribed, relatively homogenous lesions. Necrosis and cystic degeneration can be seen in larger lesions. Twenty percent of the tumors are calcified. When invasion of adjacent structures is seen by radiology, the tumors are more likely to be malignant.

TABLE 8-1. Clinical syndromes associated with pancreatic endocrine tumors.

---

Insulinoma
   Insulin-induced hypoglycemia (sweating, nervousness, hunger)

Glucagonomas
   Hyperglycemia, anemia, and a migratory skin rash

Gastrinomas
   Gastric hyperacidity and recurrent gastrointestinal ulceration

VIPomas
   Chronic watery diarrhea

Somatostatinomas
   Hyperglycemia, cholelithiasis, steatorrhea

Nonfunctioning neoplasms
   Mass effect or incidentally identified

---

# General Diagnostic Approach

Most PETs present as solid lesions; however, a small subset will appear cystic. Rarely, cystic PETs may have some specific features, such as enhancement, that allow radiologists to diagnose them prospectively; in many instances, these tumors can be mistaken for other types of cystic neoplasia. Fortunately, the cytologic appearance readily distinguishes cystic PET from other cystic neoplasms. Both solid and cystic PETs provide highly cellular samples with cytologic features consistent with that of an epithelioid neoplasm (Figures 8-1 and 8-2). Cytologic clues are often present that strongly suggest the diagnosis of PETs; however, we still recommend ancillary studies such as immunocytochemistry for a definitive diagnosis.

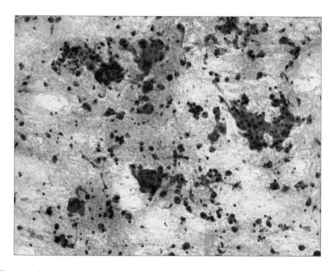

FIGURE 8-1. Background proteineous fluid can be seen in an aspirate of a pancreatic endocrine tumor with cystic changes. Papanicolaou stain; original magnification, ×40.

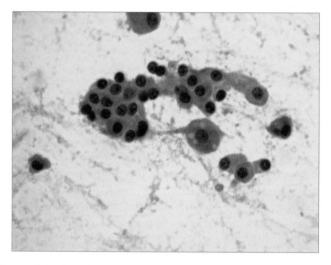

FIGURE 8-2. Occasional macrophages and background proteinaeous material can be seen in aspirates of cystic pancreatic endocrine tumors. Papanicolaou stain; original magnification, ×100.

# Diagnostic Criteria (Table 8-2)

Aspirates from PETs are typically cellular. By low-power magnification, the cells are loosely cohesive and relatively monotonous (Figure 8-3). The neoplastic cells can be arranged singly, in clusters of varying sizes, in large flat sheets (Figure 8-4), and, not infrequently, in rosettes or pseudorosettes (Figure 8-5). One pattern often predominates over the others. The background is either clean or hemorrhagic. Naked nuclei are common and can be much more numerous than intact cells (Figure 8-6). Thin capillaries are sometimes observed, particularly in highly cellular specimens. Finally, background calcification and even amyloid can also be seen.

Individual cells from most tumors are round to polygonal and range from small to medium-sized (Figure 8-7). Some tumors, however, may be composed predominantly of onco-cytic, clear/vacuolated, or spindle-shaped cells. The amount of cytoplasm can vary greatly from case to case and even within a single case from scant to abundant. The cytoplasm usually appears delicate, granular, and amphophilic or

TABLE 8-2. Cytologic features of pancreatic endocrine tumors.

Typical cytologic features of pancreatic endocrine tumors
    Cellular aspirates
    Loosely cohesive cell groups
    Rosette or pseudorosette formation
    Relatively uniform, round-to-polygonal tumor cells
    Plasmacytoid cells
    Salt-and-pepper chromatin
Less frequent cytologic features of pancreatic endocrine tumors
    Predominantly single cells or predominantly large cohesive sheets
    Bi- and multinucleation
    Nuclear pleomorphism
    Mitotic figures
    Naked nuclei
    Red cytoplasmic granules
    Other cell types: clear, oncocytic, and spindled
    Necrotic debris
    Calcification
    Amyloid deposition

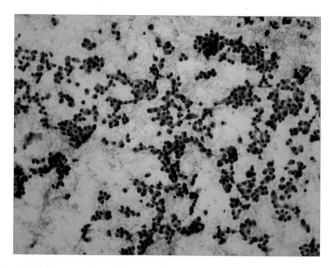

FIGURE 8-3. A cellular aspirate from a pancreatic endocrine tumor showing loosely cohesive, relatively monotonous neoplastic cells. Papanicolaou stain, ×40.

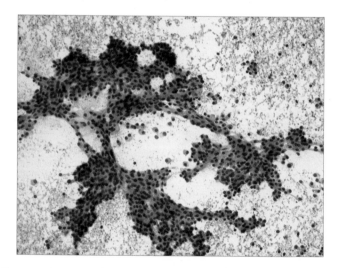

FIGURE 8-4. The cells can also form large tissue fragments. Papanicolaou stain; original magnification, ×40.

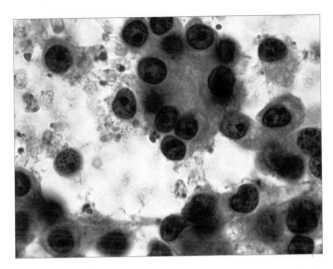

FIGURE 8-5. An example of pseudorosette formation. Papanicolaou stain; original magnification, ×400.

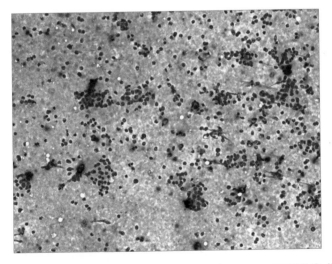

FIGURE 8-6. Numerous naked nuclei are often present. Diff-Quik stain; original magnification, ×40.

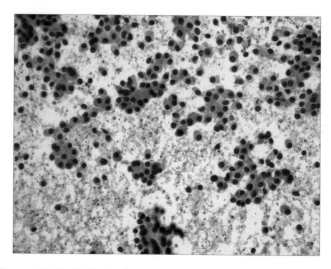

FIGURE 8-7. Individual cells are round to polygonal and range from small to medium-sized. Papanicolaou stain; original magnification, ×100.

basophilic (Figures 8-8 and 8-9). The presence of fine, red cytoplasmic granules seen by Diff-Quik stain (Figure 8-10) and cytoplasmic vacuolization also have been described (Figure 8-11).

The nuclei are round to oval and have smooth contours (Figure 8-12). They tend to be eccentrically located, and give the cell a plasmacytoid appearance. The chromatin is characteristically described as finely granular or "salt and pepper" (Figure 8-13). Nucleoli are usually small and inconspicuous; however, prominent nucleoli can be present and should not entirely dissuade one from making a diagnosis of PET (Figure 8-14). Nuclear pleomorphism and bi- or multinucleation may be found and their presence is not indicative of malignancy (Figures 8-15 and 8-16). Mitotic figures (Figure 8-17) and necrosis are rarely identified, and their presence suggests an aggressive clinical course.

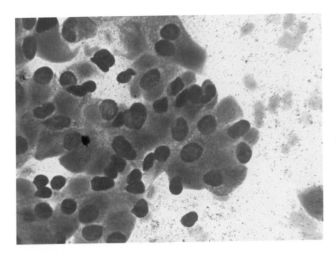

FIGURE 8-8. Occasional cases have individual tumor cells with a moderate amount of granular cytoplasm. Diff-Quik stain; original magnification, ×200.

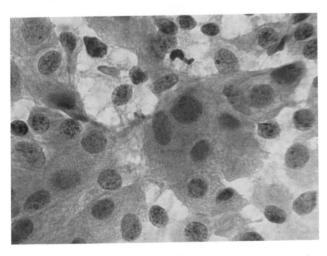

FIGURE 8-9. Tumor cells having granular cytoplasm are easier to appreciate after alcohol fixation than on air-dried preparations. Papanicolaou stain; original magnification, ×400.

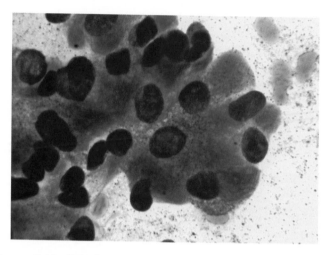

FIGURE 8-10. Cytoplasmic red granules are characteristic of many neuroendocrine tumors. Diff-Quik stain; original magnification, ×400.

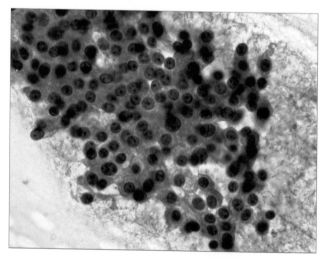

FIGURE 8-11. Some tumor cells may demonstrate cytoplasmic vacuolation and mimic a ductal adenocarcinoma. Papanicolaou stain; original magnification, ×100.

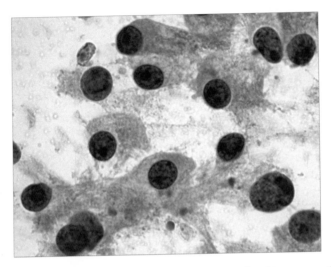

FIGURE 8-12. The nuclei of PETs are round to oval and have smooth contours. Papanicolaou stain; original magnification, ×400.

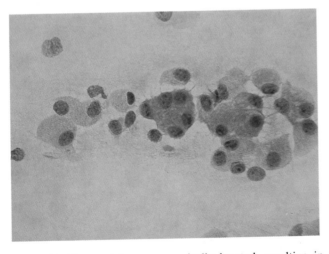

FIGURE 8-13. The nuclei are eccentrically located, resulting in a plasmacytoid appearance. The chromatin appears finely granular or "salt and pepper" with indistinct nucleoli. Papanicolaou stain; original magnification, ×200.

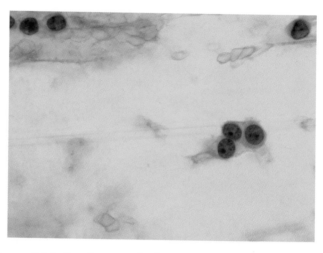

FIGURE 8-14. Prominent nucleoli can be seen in occasional cells. Papanicolaou stain; original magnification, ×400.

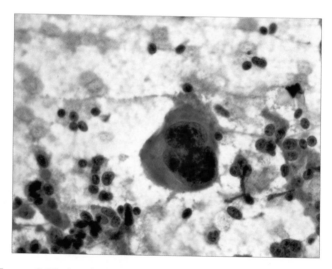

FIGURE 8-15. Atypical multinucleated giant cells can sometimes be found with aspirates of PETs. Papanicolaou stain; original magnification, ×200.

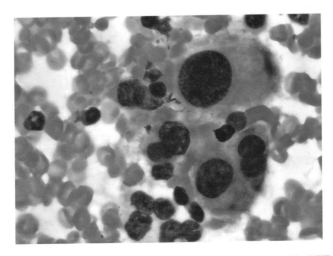

FIGURE 8-16. Significant anisonucleosis can be seen with PETs. Diff-Quik stain; original magnification, ×600.

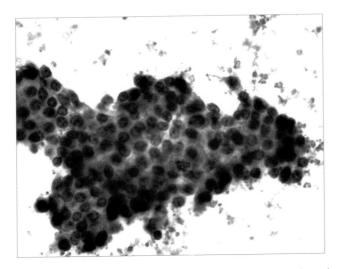

FIGURE 8-17. Rare mitotic figures can be seen in a pancreatic endocrine tumors. Papanicolaou stain; original magnification, ×200.

# Differential Diagnosis (Table 8-3)

The differential diagnosis of PETs includes other pancreatic tumors that have a relatively monomorphic appearance by cytology, such as well-differentiated pancreatic ductal adenocarcinoma (PDA), acinar cell carcinoma (ACC), solid-pseudopapillary neoplasm (SPPN), and secondary tumors that may have plasmacytoid cytology, such as hematopoietic malignancies and melanoma. Well-differentiated PDAs will yield two-dimensional sheets of cohesive cells that often demonstrate a characteristic "drunken honeycomb" appearance. Individual cells display more conspicuous nuclear atypia and mitotic figures and necrosis are more frequent. Rosette or pseudorosette formation seen with samples from PETs may resemble the acinar formation that is seen with samples of ACC. Neoplastic acinar cells, however, have more coarsely granular, basophilic cytoplasm and prominent nucleoli while lacking the typical "salt-and-pepper" chromatin of endocrine cells. Solid-pseudopapillary neoplasms are also composed of monotonous cells but most frequently occur in young to middle-aged women and will demonstrate branching papillary structures with fibrovascular cores and metachromatic hyaline globules in cytologic preparations.

The presence of plasmactyoid cells in a pancreatic aspirate is usually indicative of an endocrine tumor; however, plasma cell dyscrasias (Figure 8-18), other hematopoeitic malignancies, and metastatic melanomas (Figure 8-19) can all involve the pancreas and may show predominantly loosely cohesive

TABLE 8-3. Differential diagnosis of pancreatic endocrine tumors.

Monotonous population of cells
    Well-differentiated pancreatic ductal carcinoma
    Acinar cell carcinoma
    Solid-pseudopapillary neoplasm
Plasmacytoid cells
    Plasma cell dyscrasias or other hematopoietic malignancies
    Malignant melanoma
"Islet cell hyperplasia"

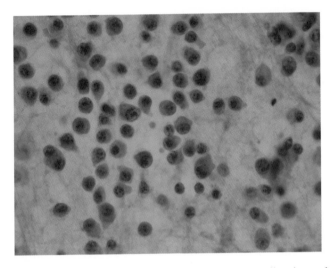

FIGURE 8-18. Without patient history or ancillary studies, it can be very difficult to distinguish aspirates of a plasmacytomas from PETs. Papanicolaou stain; original magnification, ×100.

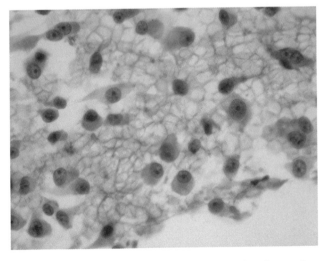

FIGURE 8-19. The presence of prominent nucleoli and conspicuous atypia would lead one to favor a diagnosis of melanoma despite the plasmacytoid appearance of these melanoma cells. Papanicolaou stain; original magnification, ×100.

and/or isolated plasmacytoid cells. The knowledge of a prior malignancy and the use of ancillary studies can be helpful for distinguishing these tumors.

The cytologic findings of "islet cell hyperplasia" are essentially indistinguishable from those of PETs. Clinical findings that favor the former include the presence of predisposing factors such as diabetes mellitus, chronic pancreatitis, Beckwith–Wiedemann syndrome, and small size of the lesion itself. Aspirates from such cases usually exhibit a lower cellularity with intermixed pancreatic ductal and acinar cells.

## Ancillary Studies (Table 8-4)

Pancreatic endocrine tumors react strongly and diffusely with antibodies to neuroendocrine antigens, such as neuron-specific enolase (NSE), chromogranin A, synaptophysin, and CD56 (Figure 8-20). Most of these tumors are immunoreactive with antibodies to CAM 5.2, but only half react with antibodies to AE1/AE3. Staining for cytokeratins 7 or 20 is usually negative. Immunocytochemistry can also be used for demonstrating peptide hormones produced by individual tumors; however, serum enzymatic assays are more sensitive. Tumors are only classified as functioning when a distinct clinical syndrome is present.

Immunocytochemistry is also helpful for differentiating PETs from other lesions that have plasmacytoid appearance.

TABLE 8-4. Immunoprofile of pancreatic endocrine tumors.

Neuron-specific enolase +
Chromogranin A +
Synaptophysin +
CD56 +
CAM5.2 +
AE1/AE3 (variable)
CK7 –
CK20 –

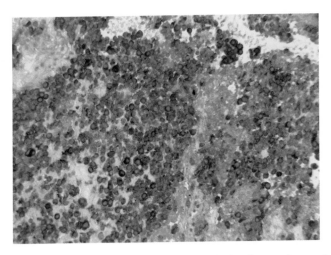

FIGURE 8-20. The tumor cells in this cell block of an aspirate of a PET are strongly immunoreactive with antibodies to synaptophysin. Original magnification, ×100.

Unlike melanoma, PETs will not react with antibodies to S100 or other more specific markers of melanoma, such as HMB45 and MART-1. They will also not react with antibodies to leukocytic or plasmacytic antigens such as CD45 or CD138.

Some investigators have attempted to use ancillary studies to predict biologic behavior of PETs based on histologic specimens. Similar attempts have been made with cytology preparations. For example, some authors have suggested measuring cellular proliferation with Ki-67 immunostaining and have noted that tumors with high staining indices have a greater likelihood of behaving malignantly. The clinical utility of this assay has not yet been validated in well-controlled prospective studies. In addition, we do not suggest using immunocytochemistry to determine which particular peptide hormones are produced for the purpose of predicting the biologic behavior.

# Clinical Management and Prognosis

Surgery is indicated for PETs, sometimes even in the face of liver metastases. Surgery with or without radiofrequency ablation for treatment of liver metastases may improve quality of life by reducing symptoms and may even increase overall survival. Systemic medical therapy, consisting of chemotherapy, tumor-targeted radioactive treatment, somatostatin analogues, and alpha-interferon, is also available for palliation and control of hormonal symptoms.

Overall, the 5- and 10-year survival rates for patients with PETs are 65% and 50%, respectively. Patients with complete tumor resection/ablation and those with insulinomas have excellent 5- and 10-year survival rates, in the range of 90%.

## Suggested Reading

Bret PM, Nicolet V, Labadie M. Percutaneous fine-needle aspiration biopsy of the pancreas. Diagn Cytopathol 1986;2:221–227.

Gala I, Atkinson BF, Nicosia RF, Hermann GA. Fine-needle aspiration cytology of idiopathic pancreatic islet cell adenosis. Diagn Cytopathol 1993;9:453–456.

Gu M, Ghafari S, Lin F, Ramzy I. Cytological diagnosis of endocrine tumors of the pancreas by endoscopic ultrasound-guided fine-needle aspiration biopsy. Diagn Cytopathol 2005;32:204–210.

Nguyen GK. Cytology of hyperplastic endocrine cells of the pancreas in fine needle aspiration biopsy. Acta Cytol 1984; 28:499–502.

Noone TC, Hosey J, Firat Z, Semelka RC. Imaging and localization of islet-cell tumours of the pancreas on CT and MRI. Best Pract Res Clin Endocrinol Metab 2005;19:195–211.

Pelosi G, Bresaola E, Bogina G, et al. Endocrine tumors of the pancreas: Ki-67 immunoreactivity on paraffin sections is an independent predictor for malignancy: a comparative study with proliferating-cell nuclear antigen and progesterone receptor protein immunostaining, mitotic index, and other clinicopathologic variables. Hum Pathol 1996;27:1124–1134.

Solica E, Capella C, Kloppel G. Tumors of the pancreas, Vol. 20. 3rd ed. Washington DC: Armed Forces Institue of Pathology; 1997.

# 9
# Cystic Mucus-Producing Neoplasia: Intraductal Papillary Mucinous Neoplasms and Mucinous Cystic Neoplasms

Intraductal papillary mucinous neoplasms (IPMNs) and mucinous cystic neoplasms (MCNs) are pancreatic epithelial neoplasms that produce abundant extracellular mucus. Both appear cystic on radiologic imaging. Both tumors may potentially develop invasive malignancies. In addition, it is estimated that, when identified, up to 30% of such lesions may harbor concurrent invasive malignancy that will not be identified until resection. Therefore, the current dogma favors surgical resection of many of these tumors when possible.

Until recently, both tumors were believed to be rare. The more frequent use and improved sensitivity of diagnostic imaging, however, has led to an increased detection of these lesions. Based on the authors' experience, over 10% of pancreatic fine needle aspiration (FNA) biopsies are from cystic mucus-producing neoplasms.

The clinical and histologic findings of IPMNs and MCNs are summarized in Table 9-1. Whereas IPMNs occur in both sexes and generally in elderly patients, MCNs occur almost exclusively in middle-aged or elderly women. Both neoplasms often present with nonspecific symptoms such as pain. Both may also be asymptomatic and be detected incidentally.

Intraductal papillary mucinous neoplasms are cystically dilated pancreatic ducts. As such, imaging often shows a clear connection with the pancreatic ductal system with obvious main duct dilatation. Histologically, the ducts

TABLE 9-1. Distinguishing clinical and histologic findings of mucinous cystic neoplasms (MCNs) and intraductal papillary mucinous neoplasms (IPMNs).

| Feature | MCN | IPMN |
|---|---|---|
| Age and sex | Predominantly middle-aged or older women | Predominantly older individuals of either sex |
| Location | Throughout the pancreas, mostly in the tail | Throughout the pancreas, mostly in the head or uncinate process |
| Connected to the ductal system | No | Yes |
| Ovarian-type stroma | Yes | No |

are lined by glandular epithelia that have either pancreatobiliary, gastric, or intestinal phenotypes and can show variable degrees of cytologic atypia ranging from completely bland epithelium to obvious carcinoma in situ. Often, the epithelium lines arborizing papillary structures within the ducts.

Mucinous cystic neoplasms should not connect with any pancreatic ducts. The cystic structures are usually lined by a pancreatobiliary-type epithelium that can show variable degrees of cytologic atypia. Immediately beneath the epithelium, a spindle-cell stroma, reminiscent of ovarian stroma, is usually noted. The stroma may sometimes appear leutinized.

## General Diagnostic Approach

As clinical and radiologic findings for pancreatic cysts are often nonspecific, pressure is often upon cytopathologists for the accurate preoperative classification of these lesions. The presence of thick, extracellular mucus in a pancreatic aspirate strongly favors a diagnosis of cystic mucus-producing neoplasia. The accurate subclassification of these entities, however, may not be always possible. Cytopathologists should not feel overly burdened with making definitive diagnoses of these lesions and should feel comfortable using descriptive interpretations, because clinical management should be based on a constellation of clinical, radiologic, and cytologic findings as well as results of cyst fluid analysis.

It is imperative to correctly recognize the presence of extracellular mucus in order to arrive at the correct diagnosis of cystic mucus-producing neoplasms. The mucus produced by these neoplasms tends to be thicker than that produced by normal gastrointestinal epithelium. Grossly, the material may appear gelatinous and sticky and is often difficult to smear (Figure 9-1). Microscopically, the mucus appears thicker and more abundant than that derived from contaminant

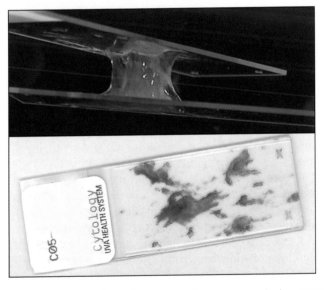

FIGURE 9-1. The aspirate from a cystic mucus-producing tumor (CMPT) appears gelatinous and sticky on gross examination (upper). A smear from the same tumor demonstrates abundant extracellular mucus that appears magenta/purple on air-dried, Diff-Quik stain preparation (lower).

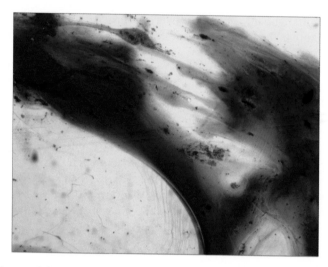

FIGURE 9-2. The mucus will appear purple or metachromatic on air-dried, Diff-Quik–stained material. Diff-Quik stain; original magnification, ×20.

gastrointestinal (GI) tract. On air-dried, Diff-Quik–stained material, the mucus will appear purple or metachromatic (Figure 9-2), whereas with alcohol-fixed, Papanicolaou-stained material, the color is more variable, ranging from greenish-blue to organgophilic (Figure 9-3).

The cytologic features, such as cellularity and degree of cytologic atypia, of cystic mucus-producing neoplasms largely depend on the cytologic grade of the lesions. Aspirates from low-grade lesions tend to be less cellular and the neoplastic glandular cells may demonstrate minimal atypia and be difficult to distinguish from contaminant gastrointestinal epithelium (Figures 9-4 and 9-5). Aspirates from high-grade lesions tend to be more cellular and demonstrate more conspicuous cytologic atypia (Figures 9-6 and 9-7). In addition, high-grade lesions are more likely to show degenerative changes, with the sloughing of necrotic debris into the cystic cavity (Figure 9-8).

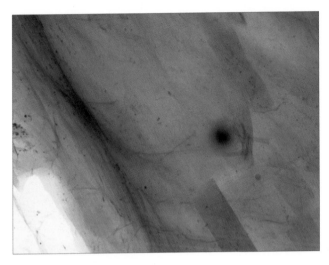

FIGURE 9-3. With alcohol-fixed, Papanicolaou-stained material, the mucus appears more variable, ranging from greenish-blue to orange-ophilic. Papanicolaou stain; original magnification, ×20.

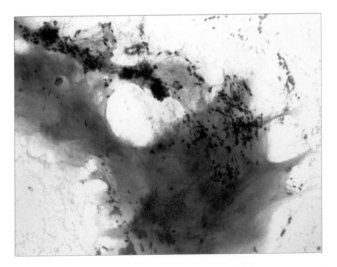

FIGURE 9-4. Aspirate from a low-grade CMPT demonstrates low cellularity with abundant mucus and scattered epithelial cells. Papanicolaou stain; original magnification, ×20.

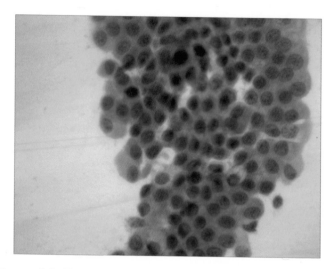

FIGURE 9-5. The epithelial cells from a low-grade CMPT display minimal atypia. Papanicolaou stain; original magnification, ×100.

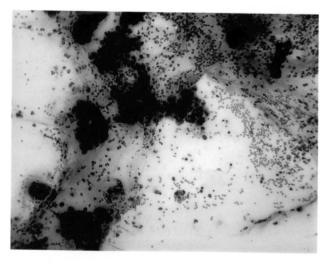

FIGURE 9-6. Aspirate from a high-grade CMPT is highly cellular. Diff-Quik stain; original magnification, ×20.

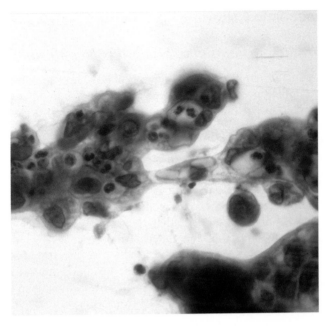

FIGURE 9-7. The epithelial cells of a high-grade CMPT exhibit obvious cytologic atypia. Papanicolaou stain; original magnification, ×400.

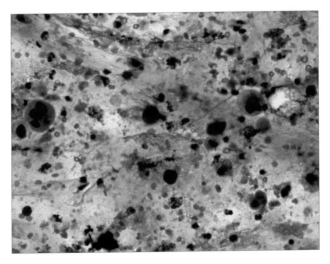

FIGURE 9-8. Necrotic debris can sometimes be seen in aspirates from high-grade CMPTs. Diff-Quik stain; original magnification, ×40.

# Diagnostic Criteria

## *Intraductal Papillary Mucinous Neoplasms*

Intraductal papillary mucinous neoplasms are sometimes not sampled preoperatively when the radiologic findings are characteristic of this lesion. Fine needle aspiration or intraductal aspirates are more likely to be performed for smaller lesions that do not appear to involve the main pancreatic duct radiologically, or for lesions in which definitive duct involvement cannot be visualized.

The most consistent cytologic finding with these tumors is the presence of thick extracellular mucus (Table 9-2). It should be noted, however, that the apparent viscosity can vary greatly and that the mucus from some lesions may not appear grossly or microscopically viscous. Intraductal papillary mucinous neoplasms can be lined by either gastric, pancreatobilliary, or intestinal-type epithelia and the appearance of the epithelia varies from aspirate to aspirate

TABLE 9-2. Cytologic features of intraductal papillary mucinous neoplasms (IPMNs) and mucinous cyctic neoplasms (MCNs).

| Feature | MCN | IPMN |
|---|---|---|
| Extracellular material (shared) | Thick, viscous ("colloidal") mucus often seen, especially with Diff-Quik–stained material. Entrapped inflammatory cells or necrotic debris may be present, especially with higher grade lesions | |
| Cellularity (shared) | Will vary, higher grade and invasive lesions show more cellularity | |
| Cytomorphology (shared) | Mucinous epithelium with varying degrees of cytologic atypia, depending on the grade of the lesion. Sheets of epithelium are more common with lower grade lesions, while three-dimensional clusters and single cells are more common with higher grade lesions | |
| Cytomorphology (individual) | Papillary groups and goblet cells are usually not present | Papillary groups and intestinal differentiation may be seen |

(Figures 9-9 and 9-10). Lower grade lesions are often lined by a gastric or pancreatobillary epithelium and will display occasional sheets of glandular cells with minimal cytologic atypia. Because of this, it can be very difficult prospectively to distinguish these fragments from gastric glandular contaminant or normal pancreatic ductal cells.

As was mentioned, the cellularity of smears from IPMNs varies depending on the grade of the tumor. Higher grade lesions tend to yield much more cellular aspirates (Figure 9-11). With these lesions, cytologic atypia, including architectural and nuclear abnormalities are easier to identify. As higher grade lesions often show an intestinal phenotype, elongated, hyperchromatic nuclei can be seen with occasional goblet cells. Also, aspirates from higher grade lesions are more likely to have necrotic and inflammatory debris admixed with extracellular mucus and single, atypical tumor cells or three-dimensional clusters of atypical cells (Figure 9-12). Although papillary structures are sometimes reported in the

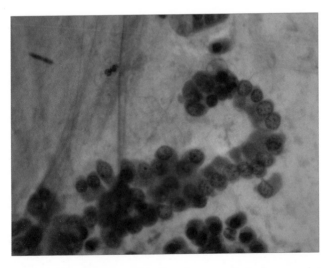

FIGURE 9-9. Gastric-type epithelium in an aspirate from an intraductal papillary mucinous (IPMN) neoplasm. Papanicolaou stain; original magnification, ×100.

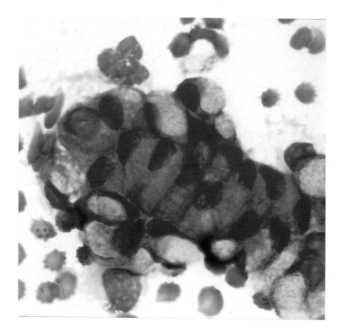

FIGURE 9-10. Intestinal-type epithelium in an aspirate from an IPMN. Diff-Quik stain; original magnification, ×200.

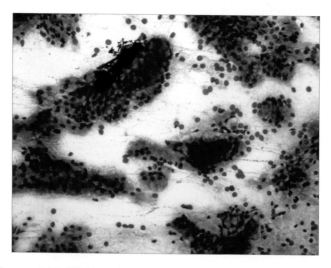

FIGURE 9-11. Highly cellular specimen with numerous epithelial clusters/groups in an aspirate from a high-grade IPMN. Papanicolaou stain; original magnification, ×40.

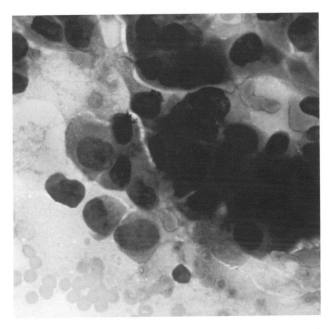

FIGURE 9-12. A crowded cell group with single cells with nuclear enlargement, increased nuclear/cytoplasmic ratios, and prominent nucleoli seen in an aspirate from a high-grade IPMN. Diff-Quik stain; original magnification, ×400.

literature, our experience suggests that they are infrequently seen and, when present, they are more often associated with high-grade lesions (Figures 9-13 and 9-14).

## Mucinous Cystic Neoplasms

Mucinous cystic neoplasms are less common than IPMNs and there are few cytologic papers discussing only MCNs, per se. As with IPMNs, the most consistent finding is the presence of thick, extracellular mucus. Within the mucus, scattered inflammatory cells, macrophages, and mucinous-type epithelium may be seen (Figure 9-15). Unlike with IPMNs, true intestinal-type epithelium should not be seen. Similar to IPMNs, the cellularity and the degree of cytologic atypia parallel the degree of differentiation (Figures 9-16 and

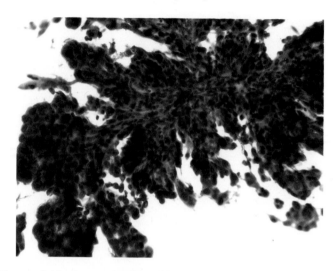

FIGURE 9-13. A complex branching papillary structure seen in an aspirate from a high-grade IPMN. Papanicolaou stain; original magnification, ×40.

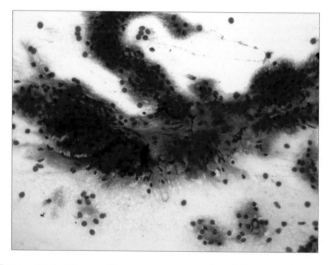

FIGURE 9-14. The papillary structures consist of fibrovascular cores lined by neoplastic glandular cells. Diff-Quik stain; original magnification, ×100.

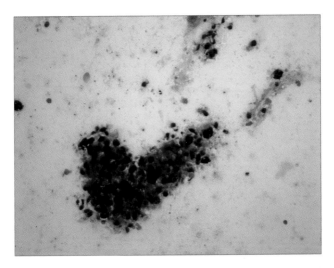

FIGURE 9-15. Inflammatory cells, macrophages, and debris are noted in this aspirate from a mucinous cystic neoplasm (MCN). Diff-Quik stain; original magnification, ×100.

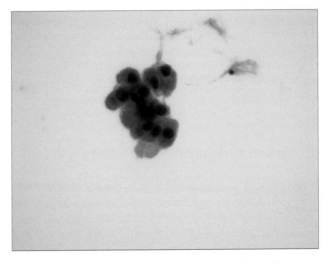

FIGURE 9-16. Bland appearing glandular epithelial cells are seen in this aspirate from a low-grade MCN. Diff-Quik stain; original magnification, ×400.

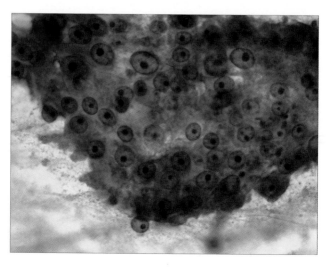

FIGURE 9-17. Markedly atypical epithelial cell group seen in an aspirate from a high-grade MCN. Papanicolaou stain; original magnification, ×400.

9-17). Ovarian-type stroma, a hallmark of these lesions histologically, is usually not present in cytology samples. Although papillary fragments will not be found in MCNs, they are only infrequently seen in IPMNs and we rarely find this feature helpful for distinguishing between the two entities.

## Differential Diagnosis and Pitfalls

The differential diagnosis for cystic mucus-producing neoplasms includes gastrointestinal contaminant and other pancreatic cystic lesions. The distinction between gastrointestinal contaminant and neoplastic pancreatic epithelium and mucus is summarized in Table 9-3. Neoplastic mucus should be more viscous both grossly and microscopically and often contains neoplastic epithelium and necrotic debris. Neoplastic epithelium often shows atypia with both disordered nuclei and

TABLE 9-3. Neoplastic extracellular mucus and epithelium versus gastro-intestinal contaminant.

| | Mucinous cyctic neoplasms (MCNs) and intraductal papillary mucinous neoplasms (IPMNs) | Benign gastric and intestinal epithelium and contents |
|---|---|---|
| Mucus | Grossly thick<br>Metachromatic<br>Entrapped inflammatory cells, necrotic debris and individual or groups of tumor cells | Thin<br>Few inflammatory cells<br>Occasional entrapped groups of benign gastric or small intestinal enteric epithelial cells |
| Cytomorphology | Sheets, loosely cohesive groups, and single cells<br>Three-dimensional clusters of larger cells with higher nuclear-to-cytoplasmic ratios in higher grade lesions<br>Papillary groups rarely with IPMNs<br>Delicate and foamy cytoplasm often with vacuole formation<br>Rare, haphazardly located goblet cells with some cases of IPMNs<br>Round-to-oval nuclei that can be stratified with occasional nuclei at the apical surface<br>Smooth-to-irregular nuclear membranes depending on the grade of the lesion<br>Prominent nucleoli with higher grade lesions<br>Nuclear crowding and overlap with higher grade lesions | Cohesive groups<br>Low nuclear-to-cytoplasmic ratios<br>"Honeycomb" pattern<br>Homogenous cytoplasm<br>Occasional goblet cells regularly dispersed throughout small intestinal epithelium<br>Round-to-oval nuclei with smooth contours and without nucleoli |

nuclear irregularities that, even when mild, should allow for distinction from contaminant.

Pseudocysts are the most common cystic pancreatic lesions. Aspirates from pseudocysts show inflammatory cells and amorphous debris and should be devoid of epithelium and mucus. Aspirates from serous cystadenomas should not contain any mucus and the epithelium will not appear mucinous and should lack nuclear atypia. Lymphoepithelial cysts contain amorphous debris that can be confused with extracellular mucus on cytologic preparations. Furthermore, CEA levels can be markedly increased in the fluids from these lesions. Aspirates from lymphoepithelial cysts should contain anucleate and nucleated squamous cells and, often, numerous cholesterol crystals. The proportion of the lymphocyte population is variable, ranging from scant to abundant. Abundant lymphocytes may help with the diagnosis, however the cyst walls are rarely sampled. According to an anecdotal experience of one of the authors, a patient with a lymphoepithelial cyst developed severe acute pancreatits after attempts to sample the wall of the cyst were made.

Solid-pseudopapillary tumors and other solid neoplasms, such as pancreatic endocrine tumors (PET) and acinar cell carcinomas (ACC), may occasionally appear cystic. Aspirates from these lesions are much more cellular and, despite the cystic nature of the lesion, show cytologic features similar to their solid counterparts. The presence of extracellular mucus is not a characteristic feature for these tumors.

Noninvasive IPMNs or MCNs with significant cellular atypia may be impossible to distinguish cytologically from pancreatic ductal adenocarcinomas (PDA) with mucus production. Clinical, radiographic, and sonographic information can be helpful. If significant cytologic atypia is present in an aspirate from a cystic mucus-producing neoplasm, we usually comment that an invasive lesion cannot be excluded.

## Ancillary Studies

Cyst fluid chemical analysis is the most widely used ancillary method for the assessment of pancreatic cysts (Table 9-4). In general, the fluid is analyzed for CEA and amylase levels, although other analytes have been tested and reported to have varying sensitivities and specificities (Table 9-5). Higher CEA levels are associated with cystic mucus-producing neoplasia, and, within this group of lesions, increasing CEA

TABLE 9-4. Cyst fluid chemistry.

| Cutoff | Diagnosis |
|---|---|
| Amylase < 250 U/L | Serous Cystadenoma and Mucinous Neoplasm |
| CEA < 5 ng/mL | Serous Cystadenoma and Pseudocyst |
| CEA > 800 ng/mL | Mucinous Neoplasm |
| CA 19-9 < 36 U/mL | Serous Cystadenoma and Pseudocyst |

*Source*: Modified from van der Waaij LA, van Dullemen HM, Porte RJ. Cyst fluid analysis in the differential diagnosis of pancreatic cystic lesions: a pooled analysis. Gastrointest Endosc 2005;62:383–389.

levels are more likely to be associated with malignancy. Amylase levels are highest in samples from pancreatic pseudocysts, although they can be somewhat elevated in samples from IPMNs as these lesions communicate with the ductal system.

Recently, some authors have suggested using immunocyto-chemistry to distinguish neoplastic pancreatic epithelium from gastric and duodenal contaminants. B72.3, MUC1, MUC2, and MUC5a are among the markers that have been evaluated for this purpose and have shown promising results. In our own experience, it is the low-grade lesions that pose the most diagnostic challenges. Unfortunately, aspirates from low-grade lesions are often hypocellular with only few neoplastic epithelial cells available for evaluation.

Finally, some reports have used molecular methods to distinguish pancreatic cystic lesions. Analysis of DNA content, as well as detection of *k-ras* point mutations and loss of tumor suppressor gene loci, each individually and in combination have be shown to correlate with both the presence of cystic mucus-producing neoplasia and worsening grades of atypia. It is unclear, however, when these tests should be used and whether the cost of such tests will be justified in the clinical setting.

TABLE 9-5. Ancillary studies for pancreatic cysts.

Cyst fluid chemistry (e.g., CEA, amylase, etc.)
Immunocytochemistry (B72.3, MUC1, etc.)
Molecular studies (*K-ras* mutational analysis, tumor suppressor LOH, etc.)

# Clinical Management and Prognosis

Up to one third of the cystic mucin-producing neoplasms (IPMNs and MCNs) may be invasive at the time of surgery. For this reason, most cysts are resected when patients are surgical candidates. Surgery is usually limited to the pancreatic head or tail; however, some IPMNs may involve the majority of the pancreatic ductal system and require a total pancreatectomy. The natural history of pancreatic noninvasive mucus-producing neoplasms is not yet fully understood. As our understanding of these lesions grows, it may be found that more can be safely monitored with periodic imaging; some authors have advocated conservative management for small IPMNs that appear to only involve side-branch ducts.

## *Suggested Reading*

Adsay NV. Intraductal papillary mucinous neoplasms of the pancreas: pathology and molecular genetics. J Gastrointest Surg 2002;6:656–659.

Brugge WR. Should all pancreatic cystic lesions be resected? Cyst-fluid analysis in the differential diagnosis of pancreatic cystic lesions: a meta-analysis. Gastrointest Endosc 2005;62:390–391.

Brugge WR, Lewandrowski K, Lee-Lewandrowski E, et al. Diagnosis of pancreatic cystic neoplasms: a report of the cooperative pancreatic cyst study. Gastroenterology 2004;126:1330–1336.

Layfield LJ, Cramer H. Fine-needle aspiration cytology of intraductal papillary-mucinous tumors: a retrospective analysis. Diagn Cytopathol 2005;32:16–20.

Michaels PJ, Brachtel EF, Bounds BC, Brugge WR, Pitman MB. Intraductal papillary mucinous neoplasm of the pancreas: cytologic features predict histologic grade. Cancer 2006;108:163–173.

Recine M, Kaw M, Evans DB, Krishnamurthy S. Fine-needle aspiration cytology of mucinous tumors of the pancreas. Cancer 2004;102:92–99.

Stelow EB, Stanley MW, Bardales RH, et al. Intraductal papillary-mucinous neoplasm of the pancreas. The findings and limitations of cytologic samples obtained by endoscopic ultrasound-guided fine-needle aspiration. Am J Clin Pathol 2003;120:398–404.

Tanaka M, Chari S, Adsay V, et al., and the International Association of Pancreatology. International consensus guidelines for management of intraductal papillary mucinous neoplasms and mucinous cystic neoplasms of the pancreas. Pancreatology 2006;6:17–32.

Thompson LD, Becker RC, Przygodzki RM, Adair CF, Heffess CS. Mucinous cystic neoplasm (mucinous cystadenocarcinoma of low-grade malignant potential) of the pancreas: a clinicopathologic study of 130 cases. Am J Surg Pathol 1999;23:1–16.

van der Waaij LA, van Dullemen HM, Porte RJ. Cyst fluid analysis in the differential diagnosis of pancreatic cystic lesions: a pooled analysis. Gastrointest Endosc 2005;62:383–389.

# 10
# Other Cystic Lesions of the Pancreas

Aside from cystic mucus-producing neoplasms, namely, intra-ductal papillary mucinous neoplasms (IPMNs) and mucinous cystic neoplasms (MCNs), there are myriads of other cystic lesions that occur in the pancreas (Table 10-1). These include neoplasms that may typically appear solid that have cystic change, such as pancreatic endocrine tumors (PET) and pancreatic ductal adenocarcinomas (PDA). Also included are a large collection of non-neoplastic cysts and some benign neoplastic cysts that usually do not require resection. In general, the cytopathologist's role is to distinguish between cysts that may require resection, such as cystic mucus-producing neoplasms and solid neoplasms with cystic degeneration, from all those that can be managed conservatively.

## General Diagnostic Approach

The cystic nature of a pancreatic lesion is readily detected by various imaging techniques; therefore, this information is often available to cytopathologists at the time of sampling. Most aspirates of non-neoplastic cysts and nonmucinous neoplastic cysts are characterized by low cellularity with or without bland epithelial cells. The identification of thick, extacellular mucus should alert one to the possibility of a cystic mucus-producing neoplasm. Aspirates from solid pancreatic neoplasms with cystic degeneration are often quite

TABLE 10-1. Cysts of the pancreas.

Non-neoplastic
  Pseudocyst
  Abscess
  Infectious
  Retention
  Lymphoepithelial cyst
  Congenital cyst
    Simple
    Enteric duplication
Neoplastic
  Mucinous cystic neoplasm
  Intraductal papillary mucinous neoplasm
  Serous cystic neoplasm
  Benign vascular neoplasms
  Solid-pseudopapillary neoplasm and other typically solid neoplasms with
      cyst change (PET, PDA, ACC, etc.)

cellular, and careful inspection should reveal cytologic findings characteristic of the underlying lesion. As a note of caution, a small number of aspirates from solid pancreatic neoplasms with cystic degeneration will appear hypocellular, and, therefore, extensive sampling is recommended to avoid false-negative diagnoses. In addition, aspirates of some low-grade cystic mucus-producing neoplasms consist of relatively bland epithelial cells and less viscous mucus which can result in underinterpretation. The use of ancillary studies, including cyst fluid analysis, often helps one to arrive at the correct diagnosis.

# Diagnostic Criteria

## *Pseudocysts*

Pancreatic pseudocysts are cavities within the pancreas or adjacent tissue that result from lysis of the tissue after leakage of pancreatic enzymes. They usually occur in patients with chronic pancreatitis and are often associated with alcoholism. They may also develop after an injury to the pancreas that may be ischemic or traumatic. The lesions appear cystic by radiology and are often seen with features of chronic pancreatitis, such as pancreatic calcification. Although the radiographic features are often diagnostic, occasional cases will present with less specific features and require a tissue diagnosis. Histologically, the cysts lack an actual epithelial lining and the cavities are filled with necrotic, hemorrhagic, and inflammatory debris.

Cytologically, samples from pseudocysts show amorphous and cellular debris and mixed inflammatory cells with numerous macrophages, many of which contain hemosiderin (Figures 10-1 and 10-2). Epithelial cells, technically, should not be present but may be seen as contaminants either from the gastrointestinal (GI) wall or adjacent pancreas. If the adjacent pancreas is sampled, features of chronic pancreatitis may be seen. Neither extracellular mucus nor any significant epithelial atypia should be present. Cyst fluid analysis usually

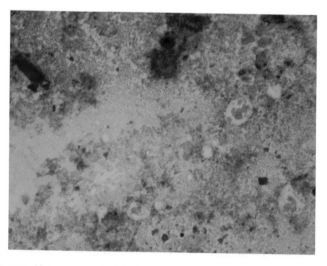

FIGURE 10-1. An aspirate of a pseudocyst showing predominantly amorphous debris, calcified debris, and inflammatory cells. Epithelial cells are not apparent. Papanicolaou stain; original magnification, ×40.

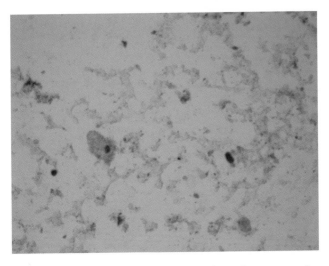

FIGURE 10-2. High power image of an aspirate from a pseudocyst showing scattered histiocytes and inflammatory cells in an amorphous, proteinaceous background. Papanicolaou stain; original magnification, ×400.

shows a markedly elevated amylase level with normal or slightly increased CEA concentration.

## Infectious Cysts

Infectious cysts of the pancreas are rare and may be caused by a great variety of organisms. Abscesses, secondary to either bacterial or fungal infections, may develop. Samples from these lesions will show abundant neutrophils and debris. Organisms may be identified, with or without histochemical stains and appropriate microbiologic cultures should be obtained, if possible. Parasitic infections may also lead to cyst formation within the pancreas, and aspirates from these lesions often show abundant eosinophils. Organisms and ova may also be seen. Giardia and liver flukes (Clonorchis and Opisthorchis) have been described (Figures 10-3 and 10-4), as have hooklets and protoscolices from hydatid cysts.

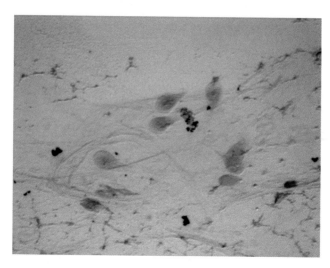

FIGURE 10-3. Numerous Giardia were noted in the aspirate of cystically dilated pancreatic duct. Hemotoxylin and eosin stain; original magnification, ×600.

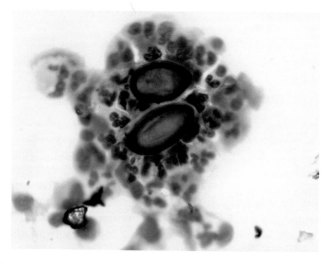

FIGURE 10-4. The ova of a liver fluke (Clonorchis) seen in an aspirate of a patient with pancreatic cyst. Papanicolaou stain; original magnification, ×400.

## Retention Cysts

Retention cysts are dilatations of the pancreatic ductal system secondary to obstruction. Aspirates of such lesions are often hypocellular and show nonspecific findings, including occasional inflammatory cells and bland ductal cells. Extracellular mucus and epithelial atypia are usually absent.

## Congenital Cysts

A number of congenital cysts may develop within the pancreas. Entities, such as congenital simple cysts, can be localized to the pancreas, whereas others, such as those seen with polycystic kidney disease, can be systemic. In most cases, the cysts are lined by bland glandular epithelium and aspirates generally show nonspecific findings with clusters of bland epithelial cells, lymphocytes, and macrophages. Cyst fluid analysis shows normal CEA and amylase levels, which can be helpful in excluding other cystic lesions (please refer to Table 9-4).

Of note, gastrointestinal duplication cysts may involve the pancreas. These cysts can be lined by a variety of epithelia, including ciliated and mucinous epithelia. Aspirates are usually hypocellular and consist of mucoid material with occasional macrophages and rare, bland epithelial cells (Figure 10-5). Ciliated cells or tufts can sometimes be found (Figure 10-6). Because of the mucoid background and increased CEA level in the cystic fluid, duplication cysts may be mistaken for low-grade cystic mucus-producing neoplasia.

## Squamous Cysts

Squamous cysts of the pancreas are uncommon. They may be either lymphoepithelial cysts (LECs), intrapancreatic splenic epithelial inclusion cysts, or dermoid cysts (mature cystic teratomas). Of the three, LECs are the most common.

Pancreatic LECs occur most frequently in men and are usually located in the body or tail. Lesions arising in the

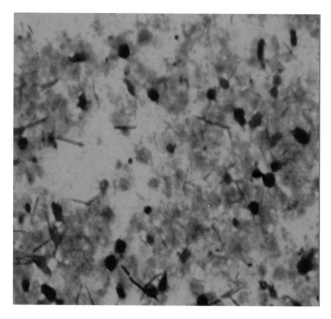

FIGURE 10-5. Smear from a foregut duplication cyst consists of mucoid material with macrophages and cellular debris. Hemotoxylin and eosin stain; original magnification, ×100.

pancreatic head and peripancreatic tissues have also been reported. Their etiology is unclear, but some believe them to arise from pancreatic rests within peripancreatic lymph nodes. Histologically, they may be unilocular or multilocular, are lined by a stratified squamous epithelium and contain keratinous debris and cholesterol crystals (Figure 10-7). Surrounding the cysts is a dense lymphoid cuff.

Aspirates from pancreatic LECs will show squamous cells and keratinous debris with numerous cholesterol crystals (Figures 10-8 and 10-9). Anucleated squamous cells are more frequently encountered than fragments of squamous epithelium and nucleated squamous cells; the former may give the impression of a mucoid appearance, especially in an air-dried,

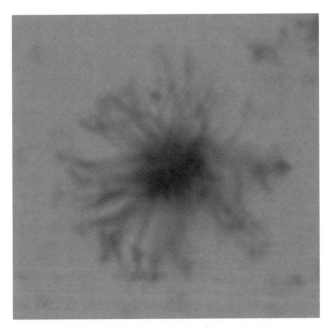

FIGURE 10-6. An example of ciliated tufts in a foregut duplication cyst. Diff-Quik stain; original magnification, ×600.

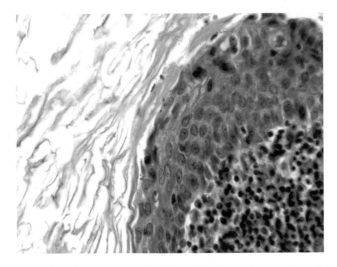

FIGURE 10-7. A pancreatic lymphoepithelial cyst (LEC) lined by a stratified squamous epithelium and containing keratinous debris. Hemotoxylin and eosin stain; original magnification ×40.

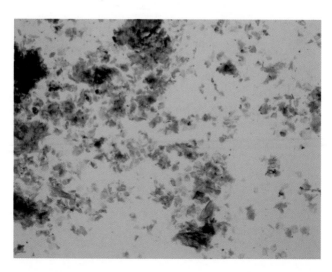

FIGURE 10-8. An aspirate from a pancreatic LEC with abundant squamous cells. Papanicolaou stain; original magnification, ×40.

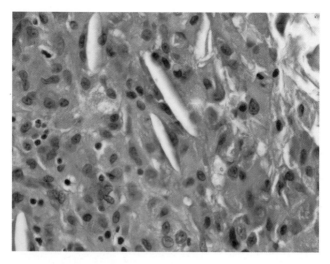

FIGURE 10-9. Cell block preparation of a pancreatic LEC showing squamous cells and cholesterol clefts. Hemotoxylin and eosin stain; original magnification, ×100.

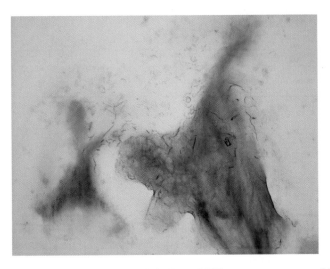

FIGURE 10-10. Keratinous debris from LEC may appear mucoid, especially in an air-dried, Diff-Quik preparation. Diff-Quik stain; original magnification, ×100.

Diff-Quik preparation (Figure 10-10). If the wall of the lesion is sampled, lymphoid tissue may also be seen. Lymphoepithelial cysts should be readily differentiated from metastatic squamous cell carcinomas or primary adenosquamous carcinoma of the pancreas because the former lacks any significant squamous atypia. Elevated CEA level have been reported in the cyst fluid of LECs. This finding, along with the "mucoid" appearance of the keratinous debris, may lead one to suspect a cystic mucus-producing neoplasm. The lack of atypical mucinous epithelium and the identification of squamous cells should lead one to favor a diagnosis of LEC.

Dermoid cysts or mature cystic teratomas of the pancreas and intrapancreatic splenic epithelial inclusion cysts are extremely rare. Aspirates from these lesions show keratinous debris and squamous cells, similar to those of LECs (see Table 10-2).

TABLE 10-2. Cytologic features of pancreatic lymphoepithelial cysts.

Keratinous debris; may appear amorphous
Anucleated and nucleated squamous cells, rarely in clusters, devoid of atypia
Cholesterol crystals

## Serous Neoplasms

Serous neoplasms of the pancreas are almost universally benign and only rare cases of serous cystadenocarcinomas have been reported. Benign serous cystadenomas are classified according to the size of their cysts, microcystic or macrocystic. Microcystic serous cystadenomas are more common in women and usually present with nonspecific symptoms, such as pain related to mass-effect or present as incidental findings. Radiographic features are classic and often diagnostic; the tumors characteristically have a central scar and innumerable small cysts separated by fibrous septae; "sunburst" type calcification may be seen. On the other hand, the radiologic appearance of macrocystic serous cystadenomas is less specific and overlaps with that of cystic mucus-producing neoplasms. Because of this, macrocystic serous cystadenomas are more likely to be sampled than the microcystic variants. Finally, although almost all serous neoplasia of the pancreas is cystic, rare solid neoplasms have been identified.

The cytologic findings of both micro- and macrocystic serous adenomas are similar. Aspirates usually show clear fluid with small sheets of cuboidal, bland glandular cells (Figures 10-11 and 10-12) (see Table 10-3). Extracellular mucus and epithelial atypia should not be seen. Because the cytologic findings are nonspecific, correlation with clinical and radiologic findings is recommended. In some cases, the epithelial cells may have cleared cytoplasm due to the accumulation of glycogen. For this reason, it has been suggested that PAS staining with and without diastase may be helpful in diagnosing these lesions. Cyst fluid analysis often reveals normal amylase and CEA concentrations.

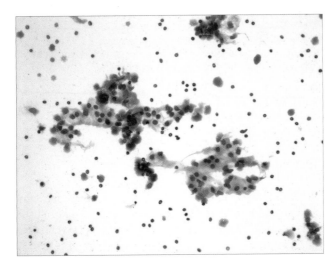

FIGURE 10-11. Aspirates of microcystic serous adenomas are pauci-cellular and have only scattered epithelial cells in a proteinaceous background. Diff-Quik stain; original magnification, ×40.

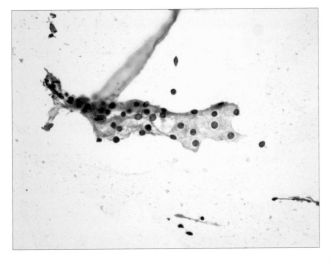

FIGURE 10-12. High magnification of an aspirate of a microcystic serous adenoma showing small sheets of bland cuboidal epithelial cells. Papanicolaou stain; original magnification, ×400.

TABLE 10-3. Cytologic features of serous cystadenomas.

Sparsely cellular preparations with clear background
Loose clusters and small sheets of bland glandular cells devoid of atypia
No mucinous epithelium or extracellular mucus*

* The presence of contaminant epithelium and/or mucus from the GI tract can sometimes lead to confusion. This is most likely to be encountered with endoscopic ultrasound–fine needle aspiration (EUS-FNA).

## Prognosis and Management

All non-neoplastic and almost all serous cysts are benign without any malignant potential and, therefore, do not usually require surgical management unless patients develop worsening symptoms and/or infection. Occasional cysts may present with equivocal cytologic and/or radiologic findings, and surgery may be indicated to determine the true nature of the lesion.

## Suggested Reading

Adsay NV, Hasteh F, Cheng JD, Klimstra DS. Squamous-lined cysts of the pancreas: lymphoepithelial cysts, dermoid cysts (teratomas), and accessory-splenic epidermoid cysts. Semin Diagn Pathol 2000;17:56–65.

Centeno BA. Cystic lesions. In: Centeno BA, Pitman MB, eds. Fine needle aspiration biopsy of the pancreas. Boston: Butterworth Heinemann; 1999:53–108.

Centeno BA, Lewandrowski KB, Warshaw AL, Compton CC, Southern JF. Cyst fluid cytologic analysis in the differential diagnosis of pancreatic cystic lesions. Am J Clin Pathol 1994;101:483–487.

Compton CC. Serous cystic tumors of the pancreas. Semin Diagn Pathol 2000;17:43–55.

Huang P, Staerkel G, Sneige N, Gong Y. Fine-needle aspiration of pancreatic serous cystadenoma: cytologic features and diagnostic pitfalls. Cancer 2006;108:239–249.

Kosmahl M, Wagner J, Peters K, Sipos B, Kloppel G. Serous cystic neoplasms of the pancreas: an immunohistochemical analysis revealing alpha-inhibin, neuron-specific enolase, and MUC6 as new markers. Am J Surg Pathol 2004;28:339–346.

Lal A, Bourtsos EP, DeFrias DV, Nemcek AA, Nayar R. Microcystic adenoma of the pancreas: clinical, radiologic, and cytologic features. Cancer 2004;102:288–294.

van der Waaij LA, van Dullemen HM, Porte RJ. Cyst fluid analysis in the differential diagnosis of pancreatic cystic lesions: a pooled analysis. Gastrointest Endosc 2005;62:383–389.

# 11
# Inflammatory Disease of the Pancreas

Acute and chronic pancreatitis are the most common inflammatory conditions of the pancreas. Acute pancreatitis is generally associated with characteristic clinical signs and symptoms as well as laboratory findings, therefore obviating the need of tissue diagnosis. Chronic pancreatitis, on the other hand, has significant clinical and radiographic overlap with pancreatic malignancy and often coexists with pancreatic malignancy. The risk factors for chronic pancreatitis are well known and include excess alcohol ingestion, gallstones, hyperlipidemia, hyperparathyroidism, and malnutrition. Some cases, however, are autoimmune in nature or idiopathic. These latter often present the clinicians with diagnostic difficulty.

Patients with acute pancreatitis experience severe upper abdominal pain, sometimes with radiation to the back. This is usually accompanied by increase in the serum levels of pancreatic enzymes, such as amylase and lipase. Injury to the pancreatic parenchyma and subsequent leakage of pancreatic enzymes leads to autodigestion of the pancreatic and surrounding tissues. Rarely, distant fat necrosis, acute respiratory distress syndrome, and circulatory collapse may result from the release of massive amounts of pancreatic enzymes into the blood stream.

Patients with chronic pancreatitis usually present with intermittent attacks of upper abdominal pain that also radiates to the back. Other symptoms include weigh loss and diarrhea. Histologically, there is progressive loss of acinar tissue that is replaced by fibrosis as the disease progresses. Proteinaceous material and calcifications accumulate within the ductal system and parenchyma. The islets usually remain for some time and may at first appear hyperplastic as a result of the loss of intervening acinar tissue; these islets will eventually disappear. A mixed inflammatory infiltrate is usually present and pseudocysts may sometimes be identified.

Autoimmune pancreatitis is a recently characterized variant of chronic pancreatitis that develops in patients without any apparent predisposing factors for chronic pancreatitis. The disease may be associated with other autoimmune disease, such a Sjogren syndrome, or with chronic fibrosing processes, such as idiopathic retroperitoneal fibrosis. It is histologically characterized by a periductal chronic lymphoplasmacytic infiltrate that may be associated with intraepithelial acute inflammation or "activity." It is associated with increased serum concentrations of IgG4, which allows for clinical testing in suspicious cases. It is especially important for both clinicians and pathologists to be aware of this disease as it often mimics a malignancy clinically and occurs in patients without any apparent risk factors for chronic pancreatitis.

## General Diagnostic Approach

Cases of pancreatitis that are sampled by fine needle aspiration (FNA) usually present as mass lesions. As such, the cytopathologist must exclude neoplastic disease, especially pancreatic ductal adenocarcinoma (PDA). This can be confusing, as many neoplastic diseases often coexist with chronic pancreatitis. Indeed, chronic pancreatitis is even considered a risk factor for the development of PDA.

Aspirates showing features of chronic pancreatitis should be closely reviewed for cytologic features of neoplasia, especially for PDA. The reactive epithelium of chronic pancreatitis can show a variable degree of atypia and may be mistaken as adenocarcinoma. Furthermore, high-grade pancreatic intraepithelial neoplasia (PanIN) has the same cytologic features as PDA and samples from such lesions would be impossible to distinguish from PDA.

Occasionally, aspirates from pancreatitis may show a predominant population of neuroendocrine cells, mimicking the features of a pancreatic endocrine tumor (PET). This may happen when an area of islet cell "hyperplasia" is sampled in a pancreas that has lost a substantial amount of acinar tissue. Samples from true PETs should be much more cellular and the neoplastic endocrine cells are usually less cohesive. One should be wary of making a diagnosis of a PET based on a relatively less cellular sample.

# Diagnostic Criteria

## Acute Pancreatitis

Aspirates from acute pancreatitis usually show abundant acute inflammation with or without evidence of fat necrosis and hemorrhage (Table 11-1). Epithelial cells, when present, may show severe cytologic atypia that can overlap with that of malignancy. Blood with hemosiderin-laden macrophages and granulation tissue may also be present. Although, PDA can be seen with acute pancreatitis, one should be careful diagnosing malignancy in patients with acute pancreatitis and consider requesting rebiopsy after the pancreatitis has resolved.

## Chronic Pancreatitis

Chronic pancreatitis is much more frequently aspirated than acute pancreatitis. Cellularity is variable but is usually less

TABLE 11-1. Cytologic features of acute pancreatitis.

Acute inflammation
Fat necrosis (degenerating adipose tissue with macrophages)
Necrotic debris
Granulation tissue
Pancreatic elements with moderate to marked cytologic atypia

TABLE 11-2. Cytologic features of chronic
pancreatitis.

Calcific debris
Fibrotic stromal tissue
Fibrotically distended acinar tissue
Inflammation, mixed, usually not severe
Pancreatic elements with mild cytologic atypia

than that seen with neoplasms (Table 11-2). The background
usually contains grungy material and calcifications (Figures
11-1, 11-2, and 11-3). Fragments of fibrotic stroma with or
without acinar tissue are usually present (Figures 11-4, 11-5,
and 11-6). Ductal epithelium is usually seen and may show
variable degree of atypia that usually does not approach
that of PDA (Figures 11-7, 11-8, and 11-9). For practical
purposes, this means that the atypia in chronic pancreatitis
shows less anisonucleosis with well-preserved "honeycomb"

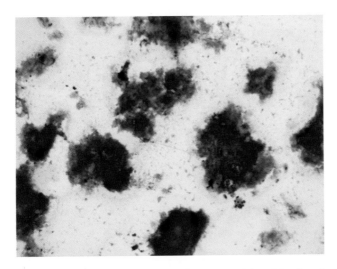

FIGURE 11-1. An aspirate of chronic pancreatitis with abundant
amorphous background material. Diff-Quik stain; original magnification, ×40.

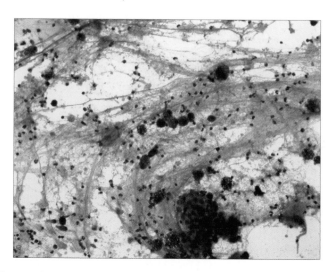

FIGURE 11-2. An aspirate of chronic pancreatitis demonstrating inflammatory cells suspended by fibrin and a fragment of reactive ductal epithelium. Diff-Quik stain; original magnification, ×40.

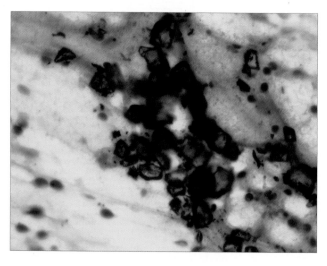

FIGURE 11-3. Calcified debris is frequently seen in aspirates of chronic pancreatitis. Diff-Quik stain; original magnification, ×200.

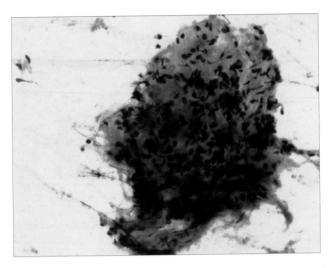

FIGURE 11-4. A fragment of fibrotic stroma. Papanicolaou stain; original magnification, ×100.

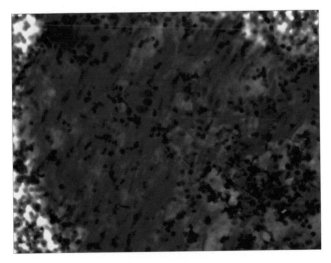

FIGURE 11-5. Stroma with fibroblasts and inflammatory cells. Diff-Quik stain; original magnification, ×400.

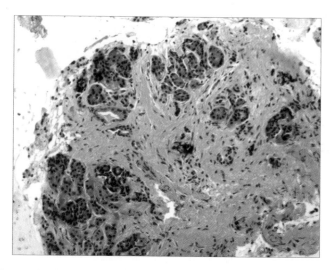

FIGURE 11-6. Atrophic acini separated by fibrotic stroma in a cell block preparation. Hemotoxylin and eosin stain; original magnification, ×40.

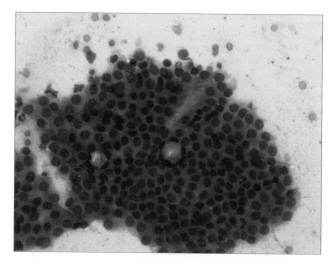

FIGURE 11-7. A two-dimensional sheet of ductal epithelium with minimal atypia. Diff-Quik stain; original magnification, ×100.

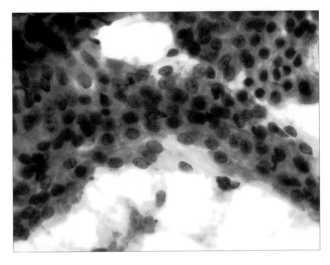

FIGURE 11-8. An aspirate of chronic pancreatitis showing mildly atypical ductal cells with mild nuclear enlargement and distinct nucleoli. Papanicolaou stain; original magnification, ×200.

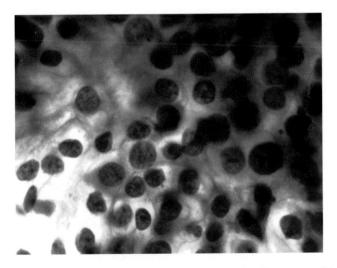

FIGURE 11-9. This single group of atypical ductal cells was noted in an aspirate that otherwise showed chronic pancreatitis. There is marked anisonucleosis and hyperchromasia. The patient was eventually found to have PDA. Papanicolaous stain; original magnification, ×400.

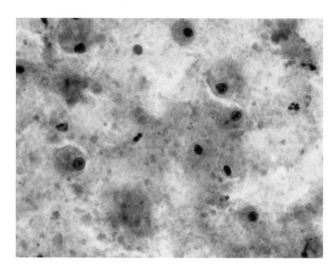

FIGURE 11-10. The background of an aspirate of chronic pancreatitis usually consists of granular debris, scattered macrophages and lymphocytes. Papanicolaou stain; original magnification, ×100.

architecture and cellular cohesion. There is also a lack of significant nuclear membrane abnormalities. As mentioned before, a predominant population of endocrine cells may be present and this should not lead one to diagnose the case as a PET. An inflammatory infiltrate of mixed lymphocytes and macrophages is often present; however, it is usually not prominent (Figure 11-10).

## Autoimmune Pancreatitis

Autoimmune pancreatitis is also known as lymphoplasma-cytic, sclerosing pancreatitis or duct-destructive pancreatitis, depending on the particular histologic features of a given case. It is usually sampled with a high degree of clinical suspicion for PDA, as the patients lack the typical clinical risk factors for the development of pancreatitis and present with mass lesions and obstructive jaundice. Cytologic features are akin to those seen in chronic pancreatitis except for a

TABLE 11-3. Cytologic features of autoimmune pancreatitis.

Features of chronic pancreatitis with or without:
  Fibrotic stromal tissue with intermixed lymphocytes
  Background chronic inflammation
  Ductal epithelium with intermixed acute inflammation

more prominent population of lymphocytes and plasma cells (Table 11-3 and Figure 11-11). Lymphocytes may be seen within the stromal tissues, making them appear more cellular than the stromal fragments seen with conventional chronic pancreatitis (Figures 11-12 and 11-13). Rarely, neutrophils may be seen associated the ductal epithelial cells, perhaps correlating with the "duct destructive" lesions that have been sometimes noted histologically. As with conventional chronic pancreatitis, a variable degree of atypia may be seen and should not approach the atypia of PDA. This diagnosis should be suggested when one interprets aspirates from patients with chronic pancreatitis, especially patients without any apparent

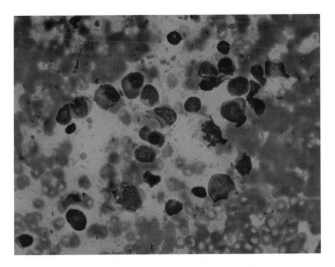

FIGURE 11-11. An aspirate of autoimmune pancreatitis with a conspicuous population of lymphocytes and plasma cells. Diff-Quik stain; original magnification, ×400.

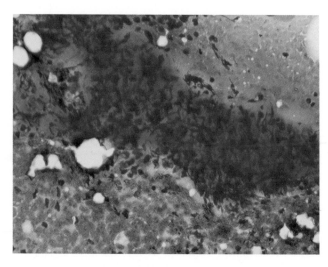

FIGURE 11-12. A cellular stromal fragment in an aspirate from a case of autoimmune pancreatitis. Diff-Quik stain; original magnification, ×40.

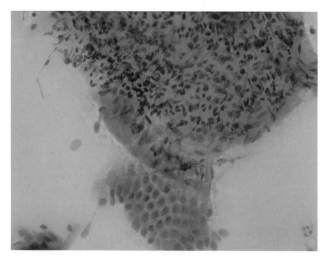

FIGURE 11-13. A cellular stromal fragment with adjacent ductal epithelium in an aspirate from autoimmune pancreatitis. Papanicolaou stain; original magnification, ×40.

risk factors for chronic pancreatitis. That said, it is unclear whether a prospective cytologic diagnosis of autoimmune pancreatitis can be made with very much accuracy.

## Differential Diagnosis and Pitfalls

The main differential diagnosis of pancreatitis is PDA. This can be especially difficult as both acute and chronic pancreatitis may be associated with a malignancy. As acute pancreatitis can be associated with severe cytologic atypia, one should be wary of making a unequivicol diagnosis of PDA based only on the presence of a few atypical cells. With chronic pancreatitis, if one uses strict criteria for making a diagnosis of PDA, most false-positive diagnoses can be avoided. The presence of even rare clusters or sheets of atypical cells in a background of chronic pancreatic should be reported, and PDA should be mentioned as a possibility. A rebiopsy may then be indicated if there is high index of suspicion or evidence of disease progression.

## Ancillary Testing

To identify cases of PDA arising a background of pancreatitis, a number of ancillary techniques have been suggested, including immunocytochemistry and various molecular tests. Please refer to the discussions in Chapters 3 and 4. Immunohistochemistry with antibodies to IgG4 has been used with histologic specimens for the diagnosis of autoimmune pancreatitis and may be proved helpful with cytologic samples. Alternatively, a serum assay for IgG4 may also be performed to confirm the diagnosis of autoimmune pancreatitis.

## Clinical Management and Prognosis

Acute pancreatitis is managed with supportive therapy. Patients may progress, especially when risk factors persist, to chronic pancreatitis. Chronic pancreatitis often worsens over time and patients may develop debilitating pain, diabetes, and malabsorption. Surgery may sometimes be performed as a palliative measure to relieve pain, and, occasionally, to exclude PDA. Autoimmune pancreatitis can progress to severe chronic pancreatitis and be associated with all the clinical diseases there entailed. Early treatment with immunosuppressive drugs such as corticosteroids may be helpful.

## Suggested Reading

Deshpande V, Mino-Kenudson M, Brugge WR, et al. Endoscopic ultrasound guided fine needle aspiration biopsy of autoimmune pancreatitis: diagnostic criteria and pitfalls. Am J Surg Pathol 2005;29:1464–1471.

Kloppel G. Acute pancreatitis. Semin Diagn Pathol 2004;21: 221–226.

Kloppel G. Chronic pancreatitis of alcoholic and nonalcoholic origin. Semin Diagn Pathol 2004;21:227–236.

Notohara K, Burgart LJ, Yadav D, Chari S, Smyrk TC. Idiopathic chronic pancreatitis with periductal lymphoplasmacytic infiltration: clinicopathologic features of 35 cases. Am J Surg Pathol 2003;27:1119–1127.

Pitman MB. Pancreatitis. In: Centeno BA, Pitman MB, eds. Fine needle aspiration biopsy of the pancreas. Boston: Butterworth Heinemann; 1999:31–51.

Stelow EB, Bardales RH, Lai R, et al. The cytological spectrum of chronic pancreatitis. Diagn Cytopathol 2005;32:65–69.

# 12
# Secondary Malignancies of the Pancreas

Secondary malignancies of the pancreas represent 4.5% to 11% of all pancreatic malignancies. They may result from hematogenous spread from distant primary tumors or through direct invasion by tumors from adjacent structures, such as the stomach, duodenum, and biliary tract. Blood-borne metastases are more frequent than involvement by direct invasion and the most common sites of origin include the kidney, breast, and lung. It should be noted that these lesions are most commonly sampled when either the primary tumor is unknown or when the primary was treated years ago and presumed to be cured. As such, it should not be surprising that malignancies such as renal cell carcinoma and melanoma represent a significant portion of the lesions sampled.

The symptoms of metastatic lesions are usually nonspecific and include pain, weight loss, and obstructive jaundice when the tumor involves the head of the pancreas. Many can be clinically silent and are detected through radiologic imaging years after the primary tumor had been diagnosed. Although these imaging studies are accurate for detecting pancreatic masses, there are no reliable radiologic features that allow for the distinction between primary malignancies and metastases. Thus, cytologic sampling is often performed in an effort to distinguish the two.

## General Diagnostic Approach

To correctly diagnose a secondary malignancy of the pancreas, clinical history is paramount. Fortunately, even when such history is lacking, the cytologic features of certain secondary lesions, such as hematopoietic malignances, renal cell carcinomas, and melanomas, are sometimes distinct enough to raise one's suspicion of a secondary lesion. In many cases, however, the cytologic features may mimic a primary pancreatic malignancy. Review of prior pathologic materials can be very helpful for diagnosing metastatic lesions. Proper triage of specimen at the time of collection that allows additional material to be collected for ancillary tests, such as immunocytochemistry or flow cytometry, is essential.

## Diagnostic Criteria and Differential Diagnosis

The neoplastic cells of metastatic carcinomas can have a number of growth patterns and form three-dimensional clusters, papillae, glands, and tubules, all of which can mimic primary pancreatic ductal adenocarcinomas (PDA) or cystic mucus-producing neoplasms (Figures 12-1, 12-2, 12-3, 12-4, and 12-5). The use of immunocytochemistry may help to distinguish some of these tumors (Table 12-1).

Aspirates that show only malignant squamous cells only should raise one's suspicions of a metastasis because primary squamous cell carcinomas of the pancreas are extremely rare (Figure 12-6). It is also important to keep in mind that many primary PDAs will exhibit some squamous differentiation. In such instances, however, malignant glandular cells are usually evident, and are the predominate cell population.

Metastatic small cell lung carcinomas are morphologically similar to primary small cell carcinomas of the pancreas (Figures 12-7, 12-8, and 12-9). As the latter is very rare, a metastasis should be excluded before the diagnosis of primary

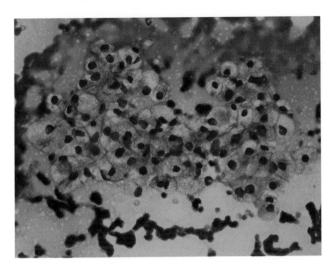

FIGURE 12-1. Metastatic renal cell carcinoma. A group of glandular cells with vacuolated/clear cytoplasm and atypical nuclei. Diff-Quik stain; original magnification, ×100.

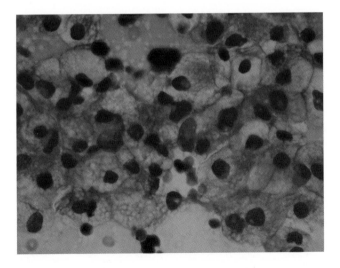

FIGURE 12-2. High magnification showing the neoplastic cells with abundant clear/vacuolated cytoplasm and pleomorphic nuclei. Compare with Figures. 3-33 and 3-34. Diff-Quik stain; original magnification, ×400.

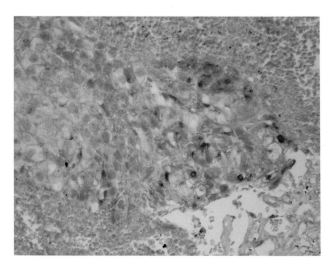

FIGURE 12-3. The neoplastic cells show focal, intense immunoreactivity with antibodies to RCC-1 (renal cell carcinoma marker), supporting the diagnosis of metastatic renal cell carcinoma. Cell block; original magnification, ×100.

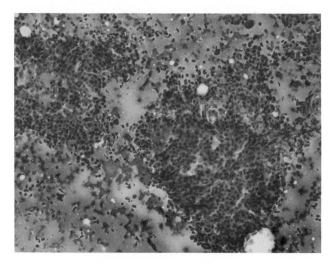

FIGURE 12-4. Large three-dimensional groups and tissue fragments of a metastatic urothelial cell carcinoma mimic a poorly differentiated pancreatic ductal carcinoma. Diff-Quik stain; original magnification, ×40.

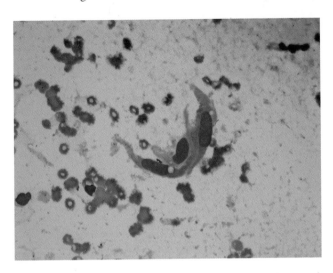

FIGURE 12-5. Metastatic urothelial cell carcinoma characterized by neoplastic cells with elongated nuclei and tapered cytoplasm. Diff-Quik stain; original magnification, ×400.

TABLE 12-1. Immunoprofile of pancreatic ductal adenocarcinoma and some selected metastatic adenocarcinomas to the pancreas.

| Antibodies | | |
|---|---|---|
| | Pancreatic ductal adenocarcinoma | Breast carcinoma (ductal) |
| CK7 | + | + |
| CK20 | +/− (60%) | − |
| CK7 +/CK20 + | +/− (60%) | − |
| CK7 +/CK 20 − | − (25%) | + |
| CK17 | + | − |
| CDX2 | +/− | − |
| ER | − | + |
| PR | − | + |
| CA 19-9 | + | − |
| | Pancreatic ductal adenocarcinoma | Lung adenocarcinoma |
| CK7 | + | + |
| CK20 | +/− (60%) | − |
| CK7 +/CK20 + | +/− (60%) | − |
| CK7 +/CK 20 − | − (25%) | + |
| CK17 | + | − |
| TTF-1 | − | + |
| CDX2 | +/− | − |

*(Continued)*

TABLE 12-1. *Continued*

| Antibodies | | |
| --- | --- | --- |
| CA19-9 | + | − (25%) |
| | Pancreatic ductal adenocarcinoma | Ovarian carcinoma (nonmucinous) |
| CK7 | + | + |
| CK20 | +/− (60%) | − |
| CK7 +/CK20 + | +/− (60%) | − |
| CK7 +/CK 20 − | − (25%) | + |
| CK17 | + | − |
| CDX-2 | +/− | − |
| CA125 | +/− | + |
| CA19-9 | + | + |
| WT-1 | − | + |
| Mesothelin | + | + |
| | Pancreatic ductal adenocarcinoma | Colorectal adenocarcinoma |
| CK7 | + | − |
| CK20 | +/− (60%) | + |
| CK7 +/CK20 + | +/− (60%) | − |
| CK7 +/CK 20 − | − (25%) | − |
| CK7 −/CK 20 + | − | + |
| CDX-2 | +/− | + |
| Villin | +/− | + |
| CA 19-9 | + | + |

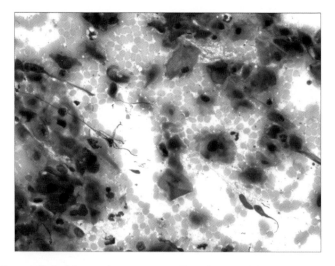

FIGURE 12-6. Metastatic squamous cell carcinoma with markedly atypical squamous cells. Diff-Quik stain; original magnification, ×100.

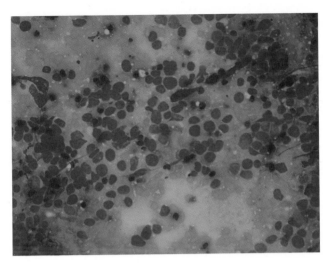

FIGURE 12-7. Metastatic small cell carcinoma consists of neoplastic cells that are 2× to 4× the size of small lymphocytes. Diff-Quik stain; original magnification, ×100.

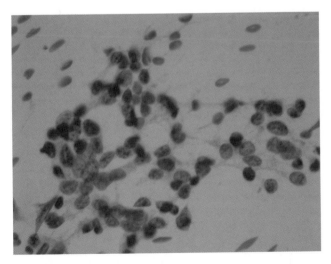

FIGURE 12-8. Metastatic small cell carcinoma showing individual cells with round/oval to angulated nuclei, "salt-and-pepper" chromatin, and small, indistinct nucleoli. Occasional apoptotic bodies are noted. Papanicolaou stain; original magnification, ×400.

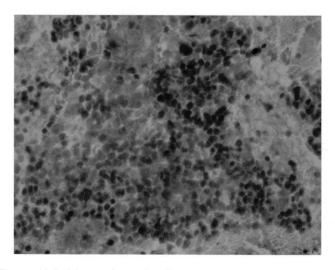

FIGURE 12-9. Metastatic small cell carcinoma. The tumor cells are strongly immunoreactive with antibodies to synaptophysin. Cell block; original magnification, ×100.

pancreatic small cell carcinoma is rendered. Immunocyto-chemistry with antibodies to TTF-1 can be helpful, as lack of immunoreactivity would favor the diagnosis of a pancreatic primary. The correlate is not true, however, and it has been noted that a significant portion of nonpulmonary small cell carcinomas will react with antibodies to TTF-1. Metastatic small cell carcinoma should also be distinguished from solid-pseudopapillary neoplasms (SPPNs) of the pancreas. Unlike small cell carcinomas, aspirates from SPPNs will not show mitotic figures, abundant single cell necrosis (apoptosis), or significant crush artifact. In pediatric patients, one should consider small blue round cell tumors in the differential diag-nosis (Figures 12-10 and 12-11).

Cytologic preparations of melanoma typically show single plasmacytoid cells (Figures 12-12 and 12-13). The differential diagnosis for such aspirates would, therefore, include pancreatic endocrine tumor (PET) and acinar cell carcinoma (ACC). Immunocytochemistry would again be

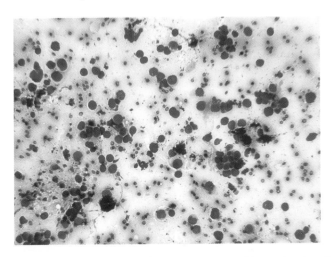

FIGURE 12-10. Metastatic rhabdomyosarcoma with predominantly dissociated cells with scant cytoplasm and round-to-oval nuclei. Diff-Quik stain; original magnification, ×200.

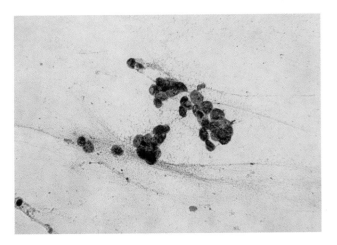

FIGURE 12-11. A metastatic rhabdomyosarcoma showing loose clusters of small cells with high nuclear-to-cytoplasmic ratios and coarse chromatin. Papanicolaou stain; original magnification, ×400.

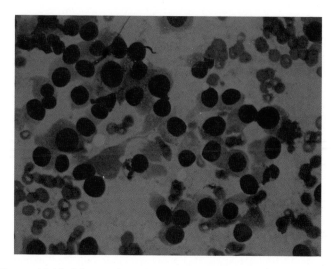

FIGURE 12-12. Metastatic melanoma. The cells are loosely cohesive and have a plasmacytoid appearance. Diff-Quik stain; ×200.

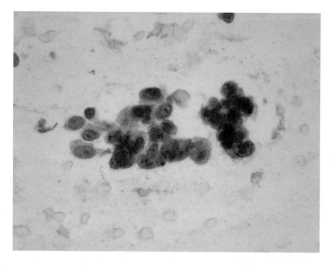

FIGURE 12-13. Cytoplasmic pigment is apparent in this case of metastatic melanoma. Papanicolaou stain; original magnification, ×400.

helpful as metastatic melanomas will show immunoreactivity with antibodies to S-100 protein, HMB-45, MART-1, and other markers of melanocytic differentiation.

Primary pancreatic lymphomas are rare and have been reported in a few small series. Secondary involvement of the pancreas by lymphoma is more common. Although any lymphoma could theoretically involve the pancreas, the most commonly reported lymphoma involving the pancreas is diffuse large B-cell lymphoma. Smears will show numerous single cells, mostly large with pleomorphic, atypical nuclei, prominent nucleoli, and occasional mitotic figures (Figures 12-14). It is generally easy to recognize the process as malignant; the difficulty consists of distinguishing the lesion from other high-grade malignancies. This can usually be accomplished with simple immunocytochemistry using a small panel of antibodies, as the neoplastic cells will react with antibodies to CD45 and specific B-cell antigens such as CD20.

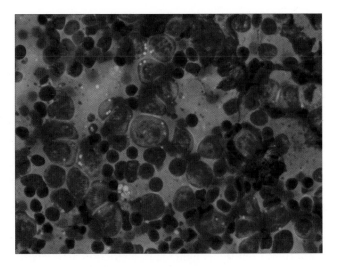

FIGURE 12-14. Large cell lymphoma showing large atypical lymphocytes with prominent macronucleoli. Occasional mitotic figures were also noted. Diff-Quik stain; original magnification, ×400.

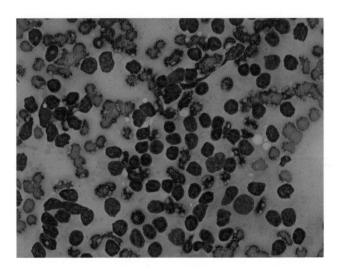

FIGURE 12-15. Small lymphocytic lymphoma composed predominantly of small round lymphocytes with occasional larger prolymphocytes. Diff-Quik stain; original magnification, ×400.

As a group, the family of low-grade B-cell lymphomas, for example, follicular lymphoma, small lymphocytic lymphoma, mantle cell lymphoma, etc., are the second most commonly reported types of lymphoma to involve the pancreas (Figure 12-15). They can be difficult to distinguish one from another and from chronic inflammatory processes. Smears of these lymphomas tend to be more cellular than reactive processes and show a monomorphous population of small lymphocytes. Further clues, such as clefted nuclei, can help to separate these lymphomas from one another. Immunophenotyping, however, usually using flow cytometry, is the gold standard for diagnosing these lesions and for distinguishing them from one another. Identifying light chain restriction and determining the expression of surface antigens are the key factors to accurate diagnosis. Other testing, such as cytogenetics, can further assist with the diagnosis.

# Ancillary Studies

Most ancillary testing used to distinguish primary pancreatic malignancy from metastases consists of immunocytochemistry. Determining immunoreactivity with antibodies to CK7 and CK20 is often used to help determine the primary site of origin of adenocarcinomas. The most common staining pattern for PDAs is CK7+/CK20+, which is noted in approximately 60% of the cases, although the CK20 staining is usually more focal and less intense than the CK7 staining. Twenty-five percent of the tumors will be negative for both markers. An adenocarcinoma that does not express CK7 is much less likely to be of pancreatic ductal origin. Approximately 75% to 90% of PDAs show diffuse cytoplasmic and membranous staining with antibodies to CA19-9. CA19-9 expression, however, has also been noted in adenocarcinomas of the colon, ovary, and endometrium.

# Clinical Management and Prognosis

Patients whose risks for surgery are acceptable will sometimes undergo pancreatic resection for isolated secondary disease, particularly those patients who present with metastases years after the initial diagnosis of their primary tumors. The mean survival of patients with metastatic renal cell carcinoma, colonic carcinoma, and sarcoma who undergo resection is 2 years. The mean survival of patients with metastatic lung cancer who undergo pancreatic resection is only 5 months.

## *Suggested Readings*

Alexander J, Krishnamurthy S, Kovacs D, Dayal Y. Cytokeratin profile of extrahepatic pancreaticobiliary epithelia and their carcinomas. Appl Immunohistochem 1997;5:216–222.

Fritscher-Ravens A, Sriram PV, Krause C, et al. Detection of pancreatic metastases by EUS-guided fine-needle aspiration. Gastrointest Endosc 2001;53:65–70.

Mesa H, Stelow EB, Stanley MW, et al. Diagnosis of nonprimary pancreatic neoplasms by endoscopic ultrasound-guided fine-needle aspiration. Diagn Cytopathol 2004;31:313–318.

Nakamura E, Shimizu M, Itoh T, Manabe T. Secondary tumors of the pancreas: clinicopathological study of 103 autopsy cases of Japanese patients. Pathol Int 2001;51:686–690.

Nayer H, Weir EG, Sheth S, Ali SZ. Primary pancreatic lymphomas: a cytopathologic analysis of a rare malignancy. Cancer 2004;102: 315–321.

Sperti C, Pasquali C, Liessi G, et al. Pancreatic resection for metastatic tumors to the pancreas. J Surg Oncol 2003;83: 161–166.

# Index